Forget Me Not

THE SPIRITUAL CARE OF PEOPLE OF PEOPLE WITH ALZHEIMER'S

by
Deborah Everett, MTS

Distributed by: The Word Circus
A Subsidiary of Odvod Holdings Ltd.
Order *Forget Me Not* From: **The Word Circus**
10978 - 123 St. NW, Edmonton, AB T5M 0E2
Phone: (780) 477-7112 Fax: (780) 701-0117
e-mail: deborah@thewordcircus.com

Copyright © 1996 Deborah Everett
Distributed by: The Word Circus
A Subsidiary of Odvod Holdings Ltd.
Forget Me Not, c/o The Word Circus
10978 - 123 St. NW, Edmonton, AB T5M OE2
Phone: (780) 477-7112 Fax: (780) 701-0117
e-mail: deborah@thewordcircus.com
Forget me Not: The Spiritual Care of People With Alzheimer's
ISBN 0-9680466-0-6

Canadian Cataloguing in Publication Data:

Everett, Deborah, 1951 -
Forget me not: the spiritual care of people with Alzheimer's

Includes bibliographical references.
ISBN 0-9680466-0-6

1. Alzheimer's disease - Patients - Religious life.
2. Pastoral medicine.
3. Caregivers - Religious life.
4. Alzheimer's disease - Religious aspects.
  I. Title.

BV4335.E94 1996   259'.4   C96-900117-7

Address enquiries to: DEBORAH EVERETT
Forget Me Not, c/o The Word Circus
10978 - 123 St. NW, Edmonton, AB T5M OE2
Phone: (780) 477-7112 Fax: (780) 701-0117
e-mail: deborah@thewordcircus.com

Grateful acknowledgement is made for permission to reproduce the following:

Endings, by Lynn Kozma

Hazel, by Linda Long

Excerpts from the book, *It All Begins With Hope*, by Ronna Jevne, Copyright © 1991,
LuraMedia. Reprinted by permission of LuraMedia Inc., San Diego, California.

PRODUCTION TEAM:

EDITOR:	Deborah Lawson Chubb
DESIGN & LAYOUT:	Randy Hayashi, Inkwell Press Ltd.
CHAPTER LOGO:	Shannon Culberson
COVER PHOTOS:	*Grammie McCloskey*, Supplied by Deborah Everett
	Forget Me Not *(Myosotis)*, By Akemi Matsubuchi
	(Used by permission, Hole's Greenhouses &
	Gardens Ltd. St. Albert, Alberta)

Printed in Canada

ACKNOWLEDGEMENTS

To the residents and families who graciously allowed me to be a part of their lives, and have given permission for their stories to be a part of this book, my profound thanks. To protect the privacy of those who have allowed me to share their lives with the reader, names of individuals have been changed, and some specific details of their stories may have been altered.

It has been my good fortune to have, as teacher and mentor, Dr. Fran Hare. For her encouragement in my growth as a woman and her enthusiasm for my chosen Master's thesis topic, from which this book derives, my thanks. For her endless grace and patience, demonstrated throughout this venture, my deep gratitude.

Special thanks to Sue Gamble, librarian at the Edmonton General Hospital, who worked tirelessly in searching the computer library for the latest in research material.

To my editor, Deborah Lawson Chubb, who gently guided the transformation of my thesis into book form, my special thanks. Deborah skilfully organized the text and used her knowledge of grammar and correct usage to bring greater clarity and readability. She has been enormously helpful.

To my chaplain colleagues and friends I owe special gratitude for their observations, support and prayers.

Bible references and scripture quotations have been taken from various translations or paraphrases of the Old Testament and the New Testament.

DEDICATION

M y interest and work in the area of spiritual care for those suffering from dementia was inspired by my grandmother, Lois McCloskey. Although she battled this affliction for many years, her entire life was one of gentleness, kindness and love. She was my "balcony person" all my life, and continues to cheer me on in spirit, though she has died.

This book is lovingly dedicated to her memory.

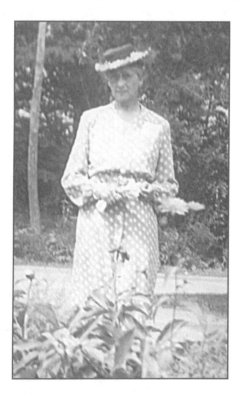

LOIS McCLOSKEY
(Nov. 27, 1890 - Nov. 12, 1990)

TABLE OF CONTENTS

Forget Me Not

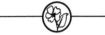

Latin: *Myosotis*

The name of this flower conveys the old European belief that those who wore it would not be forgotten by their lovers.

One must kneel to appreciate the beauty of many tundra plants, but none more so than this minute flower that rises only an inch from the ground. It is blue, the colour of remembrance. Within the blue is a circle of yellow, bright as the sun.

Although a delicate beauty, the forget-me-not is hardy enough to survive the harsh, stormy alpine chill. Perhaps no flower gives mountain lovers more joy than this cheerful little gem, whose presence tells the weary climber that the summit is near. One wonders why such a lovely thing is tucked away, hidden from the eyes of most people.

The forget-me-not is an appropriate symbol for those who are affected by dementia. These people, if we take the time to appreciate them, force us to wonderingly consider how such fragility survives the cold world that is so indifferent to them. They, too, are delicate, and often hidden from our eyes in institutions. But when the caregiver, like the weary climber, kneels before them, they can show us by their presence that we are near to the Holy, who lives within them.

PART ONE

Spritual Care
For The Afflicted

CHAPTER 1

THROUGH THE WINDOW TO WINTER

The topic of this book is the spiritual care of those who are suffering with dementia. It will not only examine the avenues of ministry that are viable and effective with these people and their caregivers, but will also consider the ethical issues relating to that portion of the elderly population which has, as a major component of life, some degree of cognitive impairment.

My interest in the study of this subject has several facets. The first arises from my personal life. My maternal grandmother, Lois McCloskey, died just two weeks shy of her 100th birthday. She lived all her life in and around Woodstock, New Brunswick. For approximately twenty years, she manifested the slow deterioration of her cognitive abilities which was called hardening of the arteries in those days. This Alzheimer's type of dementia condition began in her life just at the time my childhood was drawing to a close. Grammie McCloskey had a very deep faith in God and her spiritual life has had a marked influence on the direction of my life. I often refer to her as my spiritual mother.

Grammie's greatest delight was in serving others and being with her grandchildren. My strongest childhood memories are of her total, unconditional love and acceptance of me. I was her beloved granddaughter. She treated my childhood occupations with lively interest and great respect.

Grammie's house was a museum of sorts, a trea-sure-house of relics, full of mysterious and wonderful things. I spent many days and nights there with her, as she reminisced about times past.

When cognitive deterioration began in her life, I had little understanding of the real ramifications of this disease process. It filled me with sadness and loss to see the Grammie I knew fade away into a stranger.

I often pondered the connection between her body and spirit. Because I was helpless to know how to com-municate with her in the later stages, I wondered about her relationship with God. Could Grammie even par-ticipate in a relationship with the Holy? Near the end of her life, she hardly knew her own children by name, leading me to struggle with the irrational fear that she was separated from God.

As Grammie's dementia advanced, my questions increased. At the time of my marriage in 1972 I was amused, but also extremely perplexed, when she came to the wedding wearing black. Taking my hand in the receiving line, she said very sadly, "You poor thing!" I also wondered what was the significance of her always wanting to have her purse with her in her last years in the nursing home. Did it symbolize her need for inde-pendence? Was it her way of denying the fact that she was no longer able to live in her home of many years, which was directly across the street from the nursing home? She had formerly carried her purse only when she went to town or to visit. Perhaps it was symbolic of her wish to hold on to her identity? Most people pon-der such unanswerable questions when their loved ones are afflicted with dementia.

In my research, much to my surprise, I came upon an article written by an American music therapist working with the cognitively impaired, whose name is also Lois McCloskey. Synchronicity to be sure - a meaningful coincidence that brought a smile to my face. My active imagination could picture Grammie McCloskey herself urging me on in my research.

The second facet of my interest is professional. I am a staff chaplain at the Edmonton General Hospital, of the Caritas Health Group. Until recently it has been a combination of geriatric rehabilitation services and long term care, with approximately 500 residents and patients. Restructuring of the health care system in Alberta will change the institution into a long term care facility housing about 300 residents. We also have a locked cognitive support unit for those whose dementia creates a safety risk due to their wandering behaviours.

It is my first priority to provide the most effective spiritual care possible to these people. Such care is recognized as having to take a different form than that which is commonly accepted as appropriate for the average person. Since little research has been done in this area, I focused specifically on understanding the experiences of the affected and their caregivers, rather than just measuring them. My aim has been to discover the best way to minister to these cognitively impaired residents.

Another reason for my interest in this topic is my curiosity to discover whether there are implications from this research that can inform us as to how the spiritual needs of all people can be better met. Can the cognitively impaired person show us a broader vision of spirituality, venturing beyond the intellect to include the physical and emotional? Matthew Fox speaks of a sensual spirituality.[1] From the outset of my research, I have wondered whether a creative approach to ministry could increase the quality of life tremendously, not only for those with dementia, but for us all.

As is always the case, this book has been shaped and influenced not only by research, study and observation, but also by the realities of my life as a white woman of Anglo-Saxon background. My own personal faith heritage is as a Protestant Christian and thus my theological reflections will reflect that background. To encompass all the major spiritual traditions, and explore how the spiritual care of those affected by dementia could proceed from these traditions, would call for a much larger book than this one. I believe, however, that since human love and caring know no boundaries, the theme of this book could encompass any faith tradition.

It is impossible to measure scientifically how much the quality of life for those affected by dementia is improved by appropriate spiritual care. But the personal and professional observations of a wide variety of primary caregivers can lead to some confident conclusions, which I have tried to faithfully present in these pages.

I am deeply concerned about the marginalization of those who suffer from dementia. This is a justice issue. Societal overemphasis on the importance of the intellect, to the exclusion of other aspects of personhood, impoverishes our world. Can we learn to treat people as subjects and not objects, no matter what their intellectual capacity?

The connection between body and spirit is a mysterious one. Mental deterioration allows us a window to explore this connection. An image might be helpful in describing how I believe this happens. The season of winter is often disliked by those who live in northern climates. However, winter reveals things that summer cannot. The summer of life is full of clutter, ridden with the details of daily life over which we feel compelled to exercise control. But in the winter we can see farther. The air is clearer. We can walk in places that are inaccessible in summer. This book will help us walk through the winter of life as experienced by people with dementia. In them, we may find revelations not available through people who are in full control of all their faculties.

CHAPTER 2

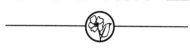

THE NATURE OF DEMENTIA

"Dementia is a harsh winter."
Deborah Everett

Forgetting. Confusion. Each of us knows the frustration of not being able to think of a name or fully remember an event from our past. It is usually a small inconvenience in life. As we relax or as time passes, the forgotten information generally flows back into our conscious awareness. The inconvenient moment passes.

But imagine if even the familiar were to become gradually frightening and strange, the least action of daily living foreign, and all of existence unstable, threatening and unknown. What if names, faces, locations and memories of all kinds were to fade? What if the ability to recognize even family members and close friends were to vanish?

Sometimes 55 year old Nora would reach the top of the stairs after checking the laundry, forget what she had just done, and turn around to check again. Once she came home from the bus stop a half dozen times in twenty minutes to see if she had turned off the iron. She struggled to remember the names of everyday objects likes spoons or the telephone. Occasionally, she even put her hand to her aching head and, in a voice of strained agitation, asked her husband Gerald, "Why can't I think?"[1] A father, walking with his daughter, made the statement, "I think I should know these trees." Upon hearing his perplexing statement, she realized that the Alzheimer's Disease process had begun.[2]

My friend Helen describes her first awareness that her mother Pearl was afflicted with dementia. Pearl had been invited to the wedding in Calgary of a close friend. Being still able to drive, her plan was to arrive in Calgary on Friday, stay overnight with her son Harvey, and attend the wedding on Saturday. Pearl started out for Calgary at 9:30 on the Friday morning. By the time she arrived, she had forgotten her intention to stay at her son's home and instead thought she had to go directly to the ceremony. After getting directions, Pearl found the church but, of course, no wedding. "Perhaps I've gone to the wrong church," she thought. Assuming that she had missed the wedding, she drove back to Edmonton. Upon reaching the city limits, she became confused and turned left rather than right at a major intersection. Pearl ended up in Edson, two hours' drive west of her home. After getting yet more directions, Pearl returned to Edmonton, arriving at midnight, nearly fifteen hours after she had set out for the wedding. She called Helen immediately - angry, exhausted and totally confused. Helen arranged for her mother to fly to Calgary the next day, where she was met at the airport by her son and was able to attend the wedding.

Dementia has probably existed for a long time, but with scientific and medical advances prolonging life spans, there has been an increase in the incidence of dementia. Medical research has conquered many physical ills of the body, but little is being resolved around the confusional states of the mind.

Dementia could be defined as a slow decline in memory and cognitive functions in comparison to previous levels of function, as determined or confirmed by clinical examination and/or neuro-psychological tests.

The twentieth century has seen an incredible increase in the elderly population in North America, from 1 in 25 to 1 in 9. Expansion of this age group is particularly significant to the occurrence of dementia. Ten to twelve percent of those over the age of 65 show some mild to moderate dementia, with another fifteen to twenty percent manifesting symptoms of severe dementia. According to the National Institute of Health, sixty to eighty percent of nursing home patients over 65 suffer from dementia. Alzheimer's Disease is the fourth leading cause of death in the United States.

Contrary to popular belief, families provide most of the care for their loved ones with dementia, in their own homes rather than in institutions. In the United States, an estimated one million individuals with a dementia syndrome reside in nursing homes, while 1.5 to 2.5 million reside at home. Family members provide the majority of care, despite the fact that Alzheimer's Disease is considered the most socially disruptive of all ailments, and the most taxing on the primary caregiver and his or her own family.[3]

Because we are achieving longer life spans, dementia is expected to become even more prevalent, thus demanding attention as to how a high quality of life can be extended to those it affects. Since Alzheimer's Disease has an impact that includes all the families, spouses and friends of the loved one with dementia, it affects a huge portion of the population, either directly or indirectly.

Dementia is an appropriate word to describe significant progressive losses of mental abilities by some older people, although it can affect middle aged people as well. Symptoms of dementia are impairment in thinking, judgment, memory and learning, as well as changes in personality, mood and behavior.

Benign Senescent Forgetfulness (BSF) is part of the normal aging process. It can be caused by stress, fatigue or an overload of information. The problem in this situation is usually recall, not memory.

Dementia, however, is not a normal part of growing older. It is the result of a disease process, and is more common in advancing years. Dementia is the result of a specific degeneration in (probably, but not exclusively) one system of brain cells located at the base of the brain, that sends information to broad regions of the cerebral cortex, and to an area known as the hippocampus, which is vital to formation of memories.

Alzheimer's Disease accounts for fifty to sixty percent of all dementia cases. Some say it is as high as seventy-five percent. Alzheimer's Disease was first described by Alois Alzheimer in 1906. In this disease, the nerve cells are progressively destroyed throughout the cerebral cortex, which is the outer layer of the brain. Plaques and fibers become entangled in the human brain tissue.

Alzheimer's Disease is insidious, progressive, incurable and ultimately terminal. The time from onset of the disease until total disability and bedfastness ranges from three to twenty years. There is no certain diagnosis of the disease without a brain biopsy or autopsy. One misconception about this disease is that it only affects the elderly. It can strike persons as young as age forty. With dementia, short term memory is more difficult to access than long term memory.

Multi-infarct (a series of small strokes) dementia accounts for fifteen percent of cases. The remainder are the result of neurological disease.

There is wide variation in the progress of Alzheimer's Disease in individuals, but it encompasses, in general, the following stages:

1) First Stage (2-4 years) "All dressed and ready... with no place to go." The affected person has some memory loss and disorientation of time and place.

2) Second Stage (2-10 years) "I want to go with you." Short term memory loss is more profound.

3) Final Stage (1-3 years) "In his or her own world." This stage is characterized by massive loss of short and long term memory.

Two principles have for centuries informed spiritual care from the Christian and Jewish traditions: care is to be extended to all persons of all ages, and such care should include persons with special needs. Specifically mentioned are the sick, widows and orphans, and the aged and infirm. (Matt. 25: 31-46) Those affected by dementia certainly belong to this needy group. The Hebrews were conscientious in caring for widows, orphans and strangers because when they themselves had been strangers in Egypt, God provided care and help for them. (Deut. 10:17-22) Christians are to provide care for similar reasons, since God extends sunshine and rain to all of us, good and evil, deserving and undeserving. (Matt. 5:45) What we have received from God we are obliged to give to each other. This is not condescension. Rather, it is sharing the loving respect that God offers to everyone, regardless of status or ability.

The provision of spiritual care to people with dementia has varied over the course of history, not so much because of variation in the interpretation of the Biblical norms for care, but because of cultural images about aging in general.

When wisdom equated with longevity was valued by cultures, for example in the native American population, that respect was reflected in the quality of care given to the elderly. In the last half of the twentieth century, within a predominantly middle class, upwardly mobile, white North America, the stereotypical picture of people afflicted with dementia is of people who are white haired, wrinkled, unemployed and unproductive, constantly demanding, lonely, intellectually deficient, asexual, uncommunicative, unmannerly and even dangerous. If not explicitly declared to be "unpeople," useless to society and a burden to the economy, the elderly are nevertheless implicitly ostracized by this stereotyping. Society gives preference to youth, physical beauty, development, progress, control and achievement. The treatment received by the elderly, particularly if they are ill or dependent, is often sentimental and/or humiliating.

In the popular media, those afflicted with dementia are usually either invisible or problematic. One recent movie, *Folks*, starring Tom Selleck, gives a father with Alzheimer's Disease a main role, but the elderly man's character is portrayed in a profoundly humiliating manner.

Though they are invisible to society generally, people with dementia should not be invisible to those who care for others. Frequently those who are being affected have been persons of faith, even if they have not been active in a church or other faith community. In the broader context, we are all spiritual beings, explorers seeking to meet our spiritual needs. Those needs do not end with the onset of dementia. Our souls crave nourishment all our lives even as the body craves food, sunshine and oxygen.

Edward Hayes, in *Prayers For A Planetary Pilgrim*, speaks of each of us being on a journey to return to our beginnings. We know that we are dust, and to dust we will return. The iron in our blood, the nitrogen in our DNA, the calcium in our teeth - all our component parts were created from the stardust. Yet we are more than flesh and blood and bone. We are something else that is beyond destruction. This something eternal is the spirit.[4]

We do not consist of memory alone. People may be affected by cognitive impairment, but they still have feelings (emotions), imagination, drives, will and moral awareness. Feelings retain their importance and their influence long beyond the time when those with dementia are able to understand them. We face the challenge of finding approaches that tap those feelings in a way that offers meaning and acknowledges the value of these living beings.

It is a challenge to minister to people with dementia, since we must first understand their complex needs. The demands of ministry also force us to confront our own world view, to deal with our own fear of confusion and our tendencies towards forgetfulness. We must face the discomfort and insecurity of changing the way we think. The result will be an increasing sense of solidarity with those who are cognitively impaired.

Providing spiritual care to people with dementia is a relatively new focus. Previous efforts have dealt almost exclusively with helping caregivers. The spiritual health of the caregiver is highly influential to the spiritual well being of the affected person. Because of this close connection, the needs of caregivers cannot be overlooked. However, the much-neglected area of spiritual care for the affected person must be addressed, since he or she may remain in the mild to moderate stages for many years.

The person suffering from senile dementia does not stop needing what made him or her happy in the past. Only memory and communication are affected. Every person needs to feel secure, to have dignity, to give and receive love and to feel affection. Although we cannot objectively or scientifically determine the meaning of the random flashes of lucidity which can appear even when dementia is severe, they do suggest that a deeper reality lies beyond the world of appearances.

How do we consider the possibility of experiencing God when cognitive impairment and decline are a reality? One important part of the answer may require that the world view of the spiritual caregiver be that of "both/and," rather than "either/or." My position is that life fully lived is both ascent and decline, life and death, loss and gain, emerging and perishing. It includes personal experience of and with God, not just the intellectual exercise of trying to understand God. I describe this type of interaction as "experiencing God as a verb, rather than a noun."

The proceedings of the Spiritual Well-Being of the Elderly Conference held at the University of Alberta in 1981 have been published in a document entitled, "The Challenge To The Religious Community And The Helping Professions." Within this document The National Interfaith Coalition on Aging defines spiritual wellbeing as "the affirmation of life in a relationship with God, self, community and environment, that nurtures and celebrates wholeness. It integrates all of life and gives it meaning. It does not necessarily mean belonging to an organized tradition-based religious group. Giving emphasis to spiritual wellbeing is important for those who have cognitive impairment for it recognizes the divine and communal covenant that reaches across all generations."₅ This conference highlighted the central place spiritual wellbeing plays in the qualitative reality of life at any age.

The relationship of a person with God is difficult for anyone to determine or define. How much more so for the person who cannot remember their own name?

We have made some arrogant assumptions in the past, such as presuming that other life forms on earth do not have a relationship with God, based on the fact that they have not communicated that relationship to us. Do animals, plants or the earth itself relate to God? We do not know, but we have asserted that only humans can relate to God since only humans appear to have the intellectual capacity to be reflective. For people with dementia, that capacity is slipping away. Does this mean that they cease to be human, to have souls, and thus cease to be dear to God?

Perhaps we need a different and broader view of the goal of spirituality. It used to be thought of as the soul's achievement of static perfection. The dynamic state of the world has helped us to see that the goal is not just our "arrival" at some destination; how we make the journey is crucial as well. We now prefer to focus on the process rather than just the end result. There is always an unfinished quality to life, even for those without cognitive impairment.

Marty Richards, in his article, "The Challenge of Maintaining Spiritual Connectedness with Persons

Institutionalized with Dementia," makes an important point when he states, "the underlying conviction is that encouragement, fostering and maintaining a sense of spiritual connectedness is crucial to providing the highest quality of life."[6]

Spiritual needs have often been defined and expressed through religious rituals. These rituals include baptism, communion, worship, prayer, dietary regulations, observance of holy days and other rites for celebrating religious traditions and beliefs. These are legitimate expressions of faith.

However, spiritual needs can also be defined in much broader terms, including the need for meaning in life, the need for love and relatedness, and the spiritual need for closure in life as we age. Spiritual wellbeing of the person affected by dementia must be seen in the entire context - biological, social, psychological and environmental - of that person's life story.

CHAPTER 3

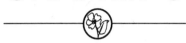

AN IMAGE: THE CHURCH AS SUFFERING WITH SENILE DEMENTIA

"I am afraid there is no point in your visiting my sister. She won't even know you." This is typical of a comment which might be made about someone who is confused due to senile dementia. It poignantly illustrates the alienation and loss of community that are part of dementia. It is based on a mistaken assumption that these residents no longer have spiritual needs, and that they can no longer comprehend or participate in a spiritual life.

However, there are other caregivers of loved ones suffering with senile dementia who visit their loved ones daily, who encourage others to do so, and who have made a vow to never forget them. They have made a deliberate decision of the will to simply never stop loving. This is the pure, unadulterated love of God incarnate. We have glimpses of this love in Jesus, who touched lepers and hugged children. It is the kind of love that does not require something in return, but sees loving and caring as the privilege of the caregiver. Such love does not need to be earned or won.

Providing pastoral or spiritual care for all members and adherents of a faith community is a daunting task at the best of times. Unfortunately, many churches tend to serve more actively the younger, upwardly mobile population. Such churches are caught up in societal values to the point of forgetting Jesus' emphasis on ministry to the least of our sisters and brothers.

Most churches have a list of shut-ins and otherwise institutionalized people. If the congregation is sufficiently fortunate to have a clergy person assigned to pastoral care (often a retired minister), these people will be visited. Even more fortunate is the church that has a professional minister on staff or a lay ministry team whose specific focus is the elderly.

A personal experience inspired for me the image of the institutional church as being a victim of senile dementia. I am a chaplain in a long term care facility, and have been fulfilling this role for two years. Several months after beginning work, upon becoming a member of my own church council, I discovered the name of one of our residents, Lily, on an associate membership list. For the most part, Lily had been quite forgotten by the congregation. No one had asked where she was or wondered about her prolonged absence from the church community. Our collective memory had forgotten her. One Sunday morning this past winter, after I had arrived for the morning service at the church where Lily and I were members, I was paged by the charge nurse. Shocked to hear of Lily's impending death, I rushed to be with her. Strangely, just at the moment of her dying, I was to have read in the church service (had I been present) the very passage of scripture that was her favorite, Ecclesiastes 3:1-11. Synchronicity again? Perhaps. But it seemed more like a subtle message from God to our church to remember this woman and her association with us at the moment of her passing. God would honour her in this church at her death, even if she had been forgotten in the last years of her life. This passage from Eccelesiates always puts the events of life into perspective. I relate this incident not to point an accusing finger at the church, but only to point out the subtlety of forgetfulness.

My experience of elderly people in institutionalized settings is that their religious and spiritual life becomes progressively more important to them. An Edmonton Journal article from Nov. 13, 1993, entitled "The Elderly Cope Better, With Belief In God," reported that studies indicate that growing old is easier with religion.[1] This supports my own observations. Those who have had an active faith, whether they are afflicted with dementia or not, respond differently to aging from those who do not have a faith background. They certainly appear more optimistic and less lonely. Their participation in familiar religious rituals results in decreased agitation and increased serenity. I believe it is imperative that the church remember those who gave so much in service to us and recognize that, for those who have had a strong faith background, the importance of God and the church increases over time and with aging.

People often ostracize those with dementia because of the difficulty of maintaining human solidarity with those who are losing their sense of personal identity and their ability to remember. Yet the Bible is filled with stories of how the Israelites forgot their way, forgot their covenant, forgot their God and wandered off eventually to worship a golden calf. In the midst of Israel's forgetfulness, the prophets insisted that God does not forget but continues faithful, and repeatedly reinvites the covenant people back into their forgotten covenant relationship. Spiritual forgetfulness is a disease of our time. We forget God in our daily lives and live as though God doesn't exist. Our faith memory might be cued for an hour or so on Sunday, but during the rest of the week we seem to be constantly trying to sort out our own particular confusions and wondering why this is so. Spiritual dementia happens like the physical disease of senile dementia - without one knowing it. Certainly this is not because of any intention of ours to forget or to do harm through neglect. But what happens when we forget? Does God forget us? Does the earth or creation forget us? Do we forget ourselves? Often when our world has gone awry because of sudden or bizarre events, we wonder whether God has not been stricken by dementia and forgotten the cosmic scheme.

The biblical stories, rooted in universal human experience, record that at times God is tempted to forget us, but not for long. God soon repents and remembers us. This is the nature of God. As one of the prophets wrote long ago: "But Zion says, 'The Lord has forsaken me, the Lord has forgotten me'. Can a mother forget the baby at her breast and have no compassion on the child she has borne? Though she may forget, I will not forget you! See, I have engraved you on the palms of my hands . . ." (Isaiah 49: 14-16a)

The Hebrews believed that to remember someone was a way to keep them alive. To forget them would mean they ceased to live, even in memory. To be cast out of the community and forgotten was to be truly dead, even if one's body continued to survive.

This kind of one-way remembering is very draining. One can imagine God becoming fatigued to the point of giving up or deserting humankind, or at least feeling resentful. Paradoxically, God has given this kind of remembering a reward. Even five per cent of the characteristic self glimpsed in a person with dementia at unpredictable moments provides intense joy for the caregiver and seems to be worth all the hard hours when that remembered person has been deemed to be gone forever. Could it be that God lives for those fleeting moments when the church, briefly breaking through the clouds of senile dementia, remembers God and remembers its own identity? Put more boldly, does the church's forgetfulness damage the life of God, the very being of God?

How can the church remember? The church must first change its perception that spirituality is primarily an intellectual reality. We must live out our verbal claim that productivity and youth are not the measuring sticks for God's care or ours.

The church must also become an advocate for the holistic care of people with dementia. We have a theological imperative to be intentionally and consistently supportive of the family members and other caretakers. Caregivers' support groups are instrumental in providing a place to share feelings, knowledge and solutions. The faith community can provide respite time for families to take a break from the twenty four hour caretaking responsibilities, and even develop day care facilities for the elderly.

Efforts need to be made to encourage the attendance of cognitively impaired persons in the worship times. It is important to do this so that the person with dementia feels included as an active part of the faith community for as long as possible. For those in the faith community, the attendance and participation of people with dementia in the worship time brings understanding of the diversity of people in the community and the opportunity for relationship.

The primary caregivers of people with dementia can become very housebound if their loved ones are not welcome in public places. Vital support flows to the caregiver who knows that their loved one is accepted at worship times. The attendance of the person with dementia may mean providing for incontinence needs or allowing for behaviour disruptions, but usually the family needs only to be reassured that they are truly welcome.

The most difficult time for a family is when their loved one needs to be placed in a long term care facility. Feelings of guilt and failure are often aroused. This crucial time is when the faith community can be immensely supportive, can listen to any anxious outpourings of guilt and failure, and can affirm and support the decisions made by the family in their efforts to provide the best care possible.

Faith communities have an instrumental part to play in the spiritual care of both the people who are affected by dementia and their caregivers. It begins when we recognize our own fears and prejudices about aging, and our own tendencies to forget. It continues as we acknowledge our own confusion and chaos.

CHAPTER 4

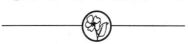

SPIRITUAL CARE AND MODELS OF AGING

"Every grain of sand has a wonderful soul."[1]
Joan Miro

"Every creature is a word of God and is a book about God."[2]
Meister Eckhard

"Namaste" is an Indian word meaning, "my spirit greets your spirit." Often this might be the only communication one can have with a person suffering from dementia. The caregiver's stronger light joins the weaker light of the person with dementia to produce a brighter light than either would have alone."[3]

I am frequently asked, "What do you do as a minister in a long term care facility? Why does chaplaincy work deserve a salary, especially in the light of budgetary constraints? What draws you, personally, to a vocation as a chaplain?"

My reply is that I understand chaplaincy to be a vital bridge to help elderly people to continue and complete their unique journey in a meaningful and dignified manner.

But this answer is only possible because of my basic assumption that each human being has a soul or spirit that is immortal. What is the soul? The word for soul in Hebrew points to the deepest life forces that course through every human being. The soul is the self. My description of the soul as immortal is based on the assumption that the soul or spirit can share communication in a meaningful way, even when limited by an impairment of cognitive functioning.

What does it mean to be spiritual? We have all grown up with the notion of what it means to be church-goers, or "religious." As we mature, the paradigm of what it means to be religious is expanded. When I ask someone, "Are you a religious person?," the question seems invasive and possibly judgmental. Religion has its connotations of belonging to a specific group with a specific set of beliefs. The answer as to whether you are a religious person can be a simple "yes" or "no."

But if I change my query to, "Do you consider yourself to be a spiritual person?" an affinity is established, for the question invites us to look at a core aspect of our existence that we all know to be present, our spiritual selves. It is a welcoming question, rather than one that feels intrusive or categorizing.

Even more basic, what is this spiritual self? I have a body, but it is not all there is to me. It is only the physical part, that which changes over time due to age and disease. The part of me that feels and thinks is not physical. We call that aspect our spirit. I am also comfortable calling that aspect the soul, or the energy that engages in life. Harold Kushner describes his notion of soul in his book, *Who Needs God?* Our soul or spirit is as personal and unique as our fingerprints. When I die, my body will be buried and decay and return to the earth. But what happens to my soul? It is difficult to understand what happens to the soul because it is not three dimensional like the body. It is like asking where the light goes when the lamp is switched off or whether ideas exist before someone thinks of them.[4] My faith assumption is that the soul is imperishable, like the lesson that survives when the teacher is gone or the memory of people who helped me appreciate life. In the physical realm the law of conservation of matter says that nothing disappears but only changes form. Why should there not be a parallel "law of conservation of spirit"? Comforting words and caring actions do not disappear into the air. The essence of all that we are and have done lives on, even if in a different form.

As a chaplain in a long term care facility, my aim is to provide spiritual care that includes the residents' religious needs in a wider understanding of that concept. A developing spirituality is open to new possibilities and new ways of looking at things, but this spiritual care must respect the religious tradition to which the person adheres. The spiritual caregiver must, if necessary, be educated to that tradition's important elements, so that what is important for spiritual nurture may be available to the person with dementia.

As a feminist theologian I am especially critical of a "normative" view of the human life cycle. For example, the normative view of the frail elderly with decreasing intellectual abilities is that they would not be particularly interested in new spiritual growth, since they have so little time left to live. "But pastoral theology must be free to focus upon possibilities in human life to its last moments no matter at what age that might occur, or what the means to attain them. We must do so without always asking the normative questions as a prior commitment procedurally, which tends to obscure possibilities."[5]

If the definition of a developing spirituality is being open to possibilities, even those with severe dementia can experience, in some unpredictable precious moments, the essence of life - that is, the life force or the spiritual. These are moments of spiritual awakening. No one can predict these moments or their triggers, but they happen often. One of the factors in those awakenings is the input of the body and the senses. Those affected by dementia don't remember the propensity of western culture to deny the body and so they respond to their bodies unashamedly. Episodes of awakening for those with dementia have much to teach us about being real and living in the moment. People with cognitive impairment need to be given as many opportunities as possible to experience the things that can lead to these moments.

Awakening is the first step of all spirituality in both western and eastern traditions, and is therefore a universal experience. In being attentive to the present moment, the person with dementia experiences the numinous in a mysterious way. These times of profound engagement with life challenge us, as caregivers, to appreciate the importance of the present moment in our own lives. Openness to new spiritual possibilities can happen, for instance, when the person with dementia is in awe of a flower, seeing it as coming fresh from the hand of God, or when the care receiver really senses love from another person. Awakenings might happen in experiencing the sacraments, or in struggling with grief and loss issues during the onset of dementia. Dr. Bob Hatfield, at the Banff Pastoral Care Conference in April, 1994, defined healthy as being able to engage in life, not necessarily being free of disease. By this definition, people with mild to moderate dementia can be considered healthy much of the time.

One of my privileges as a chaplain is to encourage

the person with dementia in his or her appreciation of the "now" of life. I have the privilege of helping them retain their philosophical tenets, such as: God will take care of things; there are others who have the same problems; I am not alone; I feel love and trust.

Much of the discouragement that caregivers feel towards those with dementia could be averted if they saw this ministry not as tackling a problem to be solved, but as approaching a mystery to be experienced. Jesus did not change the human condition, but embraced it, did not take away human suffering, but gave it meaning in terms of the resurrection. It has been my observation that burnout is less likely among caregivers who trust that no person is too far gone to experience the Spirit's empowering. When caregivers change their perspective from "doing for" to "being with," stress is diminished.

My chaplaincy offers me the opportunity to focus on a person-centered approach to dementia care. There is a biblical affirmation of this approach. ". . . whatever is true, whatever is noble, whatever is right, whatever is pure, whatever is lovely, whatever is admirable . . . think about such things." (Philippians 4:8) This means I can challenge the assumptions formed purely through a medical model of the disease process.

All new discoveries and inventions result from paradigm shifts or new ways of looking at things. The ministry of spiritual care that I offer includes encouraging caregivers to embrace a more positive world view, while not denying the tragic quality of the situation.

Ronna Jevne, in her book, *It All Begins With Hope*, writes, "I have a dream . . . a vision of how caring can be . . . where a whole institution of caring people understand that nothing is as therapeutic as recognizing the emotional pain, not just the physical pain . . . that death would be something faced, not feared.

I have a vision that caregivers would touch patients, gently and not just physically. That all would recognize that with every touch, every smile, every word, we are entering a temple."[6]

Thomas St. James O'Connor's article, "Ministry Without A Future," (The Journal of Pastoral Care, Spring 1992) fuelled my excitement for this unique type of ministry with those who suffer from dementia, and was instrumental in the germination of my ministry perspective. O'Connor poses the question of how spiritual care for those who are cognitively impaired can be done differently, and thus more effectively. He speaks of three paradigm shifts: (1) a different way of thinking; (2) a different way of relating; and (3) a different way of using symbols.[7]

A primary model which informs western society's treatment of aging is the symmetrical model, which is based on the image of life as a "peak between two valleys or a process of development toward fullness of life, followed inevitably by diminishment, toward senility and death."[8]

Whereas childhood and adolescence are seen as ever widening horizons, adulthood is seen as the peak of expression, followed by the change in life (at about 40 years old), when one presumably begins the descent "over-the-hill." The demise of our physical bodies is irrefutable. Psychologist Paul Pruyser states, "aging becomes the hidden fault or the subtle and seldom acknowledged enemy that must be refused and denied for as long as possible. The comedy of life belongs to the youth and the tragedy of life belongs to the aged."[9] Add to this the stigma of cognitive impairment and the tragedy is complete.

The last half of the twentieth century has developed this tragic image even further through the increasing dominance of a naturalistic, scientific mind set and with the decline of the belief in life after death. Spiritual care has become a matter of helping the aging accept increasing limitations and degeneration, so as to adapt to the diminishment of their faculties over time. The symmetrical model of aging thus requires primarily that grief issues be addressed.

The strength of this symmetrical model is its openness to grief over the losses experienced from aging, which are a true reality. The weakness of this model is that it affirms the cultural tendency to place greater value on youth and vigor than on aging. This model can take on a quality of pessimism, as in fighting a losing battle. Obviously, adding dementia to an already pessimistic climate creates the assumption that it is a hopeless cause to attend to the spiritual care of cognitively impaired people.

Pruyser, at a symposium on Theology and Aging in 1974, offered a significantly altered variation of his symmetrical model. He counters this fundamentally pessimistic model with a loss/compensation model. He accepts the losses as reality, but also highlights the following compensations which might be found in the midst of losses:

1) There are good and wholesome dependencies.

2) One defines one's value counter to a hierarchical status model.

3) There is a relaxation of defences; one has nothing to prove or achieve.

4) There is a greater capacity to live in the present.

5) There is a reappropriation of the ideals of youth.

6) One can be real. [10]

Pruyser's adaptation has as its image the facilitation of the person's strengths. It is the exercise of free choice, even though limited, rather than just the sustaining of existence. It has a more positive and less tragic note, being present and open to possibilities within the tragic. Victor Frankl in his book, *Man's Search For Meaning*, expressed it as having a world view that is tragically optimistic.[11]

The tragic elements of dementia-related loss are evident. But is there a possibility that some compensations do exist, at least in the milder stages? Can elements of hope be discovered in an otherwise seemingly hopeless situation? The discovery of hope in the tragic can happen when a caregiver sees the wiping away of everyday worries and concerns to allow for experiences of awe in the moment. This hope lives in the realm of faith. As Kathleen Fischer says in her book, *Winter Grace*, it is not "naive optimism nor a bargaining tool for a miraculous cure. Rather it is an open ended hope, based on trust that God's promises will be fulfilled and with a wider perspective to be given for all our limited hopes."[12]

Another model of aging, proposed by the psychologist, Erik Erikson is the Epigenetic model of aging.[13] A diagram will show these stages, imaged as a road with transitional times between each stage.

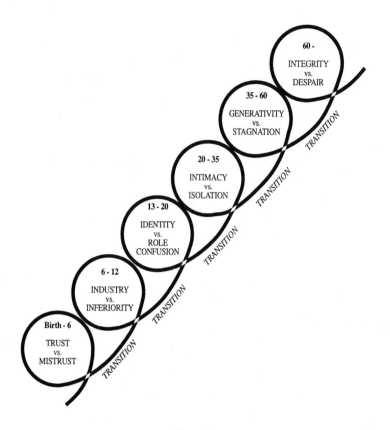

Figure 1

The final developmental stage of our lives according to this model is the crisis between integrity and despair. "Integrity is the acceptance of one's one and only life as something that had to be and permitted no substitutes."[14] For Erikson the human cycle cannot be complete until the last stage of integrity becomes a possibility. This achievement means circling back to the first virtue-stage of infancy, the virtue of trust. Trust and integrity are cojoined, as represented on the next page.

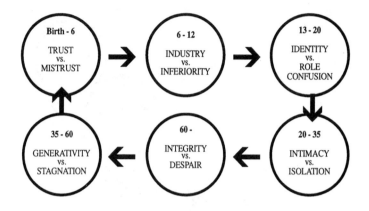

Figure 2

The Epigenetic model is a perspective on the whole of life which asserts that completing the stage of integrity and despair is not possible until the length of days have been completed. It affirms one's pilgrimage and all its stages. This circling back is still possible for the person with dementia, even if it is only momentary. As dementia progresses into its later stages, there is indeed a regression to more primitive modes. In the latter stages of dementia, not unlike infancy, the development of trust is still possible.

Because in many cases dementia is progressive over such a long period of time, many opportune moments occur in which to conduct this negotiation of integrity and despair. This is especially true in the mild to moderate stages, which can last several years, but times of moving to integrity or despair can also happen even in the severe stage. O'Connor believes "that the assumed blocks that we would think hinder this integration within persons with dementia is based on a dualistic world view of mind and body split. A unitive world view that the body, mind and spirit are united and form a systematic whole makes this integration a real possibility."[15] It is to the Greeks that we must ascribe the view of two separate words to describe the mind and the body. The Hebrews had only one word, "nephesh," which meant an entire living being.

Lily's intense desire was to go home to Prince Edward Island. She struggled to accept her life in a long term care facility without giving in to hopelessness. This was her struggle for integrity. In our eyes, her desire to return to PEI seemed unrealistic. But for Lily, it kept despair at bay. Her longing was an example of what is known as transcendent voyaging (believing and thinking of herself as going there - a spiritual exercise). Her wish to go back to PEI also expressed her search for a safe place where she felt loved. This led to freedom from the fear of death.

Another woman, Alma, is hospitalized with a more advanced stage of dementia. She loves to rock back and forth with a doll cradled in her arms. The rocking motion has a rhythmic quality and could be perceived as her way of working out issues with her own mother or with her own children. Perhaps it can be seen as her body's remembered experience of being cradled as an infant and her search for that comfort and security now. Feeling loved and secure is a core element of the spiritual journey with God. The nurses on the unit have observed that rocking the doll causes Alma to be happier and less agitated than she is without the doll.

The final model of aging is a historical and eschatological model. It places the person in history with their integrity and uniqueness. Those with dementia are contained in a larger and more open-ended vision of God's future. It is relocating the ground of hope into the great hope of humankind. It has to do with an enlarged and less humanly dependent context within which one's life is understood. It is aging in God. It is also freedom from defining one's importance in our limited earthly existence alone.[16]

The secret of caring for the person with dementia is in caring for the whole person. Care for others, including pastoral care, is a deeply rooted, universally human characteristic. This necessitates a radical revisioning so that the person with dementia is no longer viewed as damaged or partial, but as valuable, acceptable and whole - not measured by the capacities they have lost, but treasured as they are.

Christian and Hebrew scriptures abound with images of caring like a shepherd cares for the sheep. Psalm 23 tells of the shepherd protecting the sheep not only from the dangerous places, but also from the fear of being alone. In Christian symbolism, the shepherd is always seeking the lone sheep so that it may be brought back into the embrace of love and care.

"Though I walk through the valley of the shadow of death, I shall fear no ill, for you are with me. Thy rod and thy staff, they comfort me." (Psalm 23:4) The shepherd image is particularly appropriate for the spiritual caregiver of those affected by dementia, since wandering is such a common occurrence. The caregiver must be as vigilant as a shepherd, both to care for the safety of the person with dementia and to help maintain their sense of belonging to a community.

The minister or the caregiver must realize the meaning in their care. In an article entitled "Care of the Demented Patients with Severe Communication Problems," the authors claim that the feeling of meaninglessness is more prevalent in withdrawn and apathetic people than in aggressive ones.

Some caregivers are convinced that it is always possible to enter into contact, and they find it exciting to discover the means to do so. They are also happy with even small responses such as a glimpse of recognition. While people at advanced stages of dementia might not remember faces, they retain emotional after-images for long enough intervals to develop feelings of trust and security with caregivers. To discover the small responses requires a sensitivity and attentiveness to everything happening in the moment. Even a negative reaction to the caregiver is still a contact and affirms Fromm's (1973) stance that humans have a strong need to affect others.[17] Therefore, even a negative experience builds meaning and connection between the caregiver and the care receiver.

There is a circular relationship between communication and commitment. Communication stimulates commitment; commitment draws out communication. Any person committed to relationship must take enough time and use enough energy to see and experience the other person. The result will be glimpses of the meaning of the other's life and greater sensitivity to the moods, feelings and responses of that person. Such committed interaction is love.[18]

Spiritual care does make a positive difference in quality of life. A chaplaincy demonstration program at the Capital Care Group in Edmonton found that behaviours were reasonably accurate indicators of response to spiritual care, whereas discussion of spiritual issues provided more limited feedback. Eye contact and touch communicated individuals' importance.[19]

In becoming effective caregivers to those who suffer from dementia, we must not give in to the fear of becoming demented ourselves. We must not fear the unknown, or the insufficiency and powerlessness we feel when we are with someone with dementia. Yes, we can experience it, but we must not allow the fear to keep us away. The powerlessness that may occur when caring for a person with dementia has a lot to do with the caregiver's inability to value other means of communication than just words. This fear multiplies the feeling of meaninglessness about ministering to these people. When we see only meaninglessness, commitment is often lost. Surrender to the mystery of the future means admitting the possibility of suffering. Real care for those affected by dementia only takes place when the walls of fear have been removed.

Patricia Brown Coughlan, author of *Facing Alzheimer's*, asks: "What is the glue that holds a relationship together when one person in the relationship has changed so drastically?" She quotes Robert Lumpkins who thinks it is love. It is love and affection and respect. It is the strength from what has been endured together up to this time. It is the awareness of responsibility to take caring as far as possible.[20] No matter how bizarre or bewildering the behaviors of people that are cognitively impaired, people with dementia are still made in the image of God. Caregivers have the opportunity to fan the flame of their hearts and spirits. We can provide something more continuous than the fragmentation of the affected person, and that continuous something is love.

A respectful philosophy of caring for people with dementia must be characterized by acts, not just theory or words, and will include the following:

42

1) Remind the person that you and others significant to the person will go on caring no matter what.

2) Sacramental presence cannot be underestimated. In moments of fear and discouragement, your presence, prayers and blessings are tangible evidence of God's love.

3) Strong needs exist for constancy, structure, simplicity, and familiarity.

4) Christian love is more than doing things for others. It is the expression of genuine love and deepest respect and the recognition of the unique value of each person. True love makes the other person feel important and valuable.

5) Making a person affected by dementia feel at ease is important. They do not need pity but have a right to respectful treatment.

6) Individuals affected by dementia can learn simple tasks or facts if they are repeated often enough. Pictures and music that are well known can help in this learning.

7) Anger can be a result of a catastrophic reaction and need not be taken personally. Forgetfulness is even an advantage because they soon forget the angry situation.

8) Those affected by dementia remain very sensitive to the mood around them. They have accurate feelings but the explanation for the feeling is often inaccurate.

9) Respond lovingly to feelings, which are real, but don't try to convince the person that what he expresses is unreasonable.

10) Minister with calmness and gentleness. The key is to simplify.

11) Asking the same questions repeatedly is a symptom of general insecurity in people who can no longer make sense of their environment. Reassure them of their safety in their present surroundings.

12) Those with moderate to severe dementia do not remember names but they recognize faces that are seen often. Reintroduce yourself each time you visit the loved one, and do not ask if he or she remembers you. A visit should not feel like an examination.

13) Anything that needs to be communicated needs to be transmitted relationally, not propositionally. People respond to how we feel about them more than what we say to them.

14) It is helpful to perceive those with dementia as a phenomenon of life, as naturally as we would look at a rosebush, without asking questions or making judgements. Do not patronize people with dementia, or say things that you would not have said in their presence if they were not affected by dementia.

15) Laughter is good medicine. Laugh at the situation but not at the person. Laughter lets off steam and teaches us that life is not all gloom and darkness. Laughter and humour remind the person with dementia that life is meant to be lived and enjoyed. Laughter decreases anxiety. The Apostle Paul reminds Christians to rejoice and to fill their minds with good thoughts.

16) Address such people by their first names, as Jesus did. It indicates affection and intimacy, and conveys a sense of dignity.

17) Like Jesus, we can convey our love by touch. Touch transmits closeness that words alone cannot fully express. It involves a different but highly valid means of communication. Jesus did not talk to people in intellectual and abstract terms. He talked at the feeling level, and readily touched people. Physical contact says to another that she or he is treasured, beautiful and not untouchable. It speaks when we don't know what to say. Skin contact tells the truth of caring far more deeply than words.

18) People have an eternal desire to be known. Don't automatically assume that Alzheimer's victims don't know what you are saying or that they don't want to be known. They frequently understand the emotional content of facial expressions very well.

19) Reassure the person that although the realities of Alzheimer's Disease are unpleasant, life can still be enjoyed. Encourage hope.

20) Arrange as many opportunities as possible for the person with dementia to experience nature through tactile experiences.

21) The caregiver must discard any notion that every conversation in which they engage will make logical sense.

Dignity is the cornerstone of care.[21] Loss of a sense of self does not equate automatically with loss of dignity. The aim is to bring out the individual's remaining skills and abilities. In a holistic approach to caring, these people are not patients; their full personhood needs to be honored.

Spiritual care requires a person-centered approach. I have learned to understand and appreciate the individuality of each person by making a concerted effort to learn about their past interests, hobbies, spiritual background, and family. I also try to discover what communication problems exist, and seek ways to meet each one's particular needs.

The unpredictable moods of the person with dementia require that the caregiver to be flexible. This means being sensitive to and accepting of their divergent views of reality. It is difficult for the families not to focus on what is continually being lost in progressive dementia. They concentrate on what used to be rather than making the most of the day at hand. One must learn to enjoy even brief moments.

To care for the confused elderly we must come into contact with the confused one in ourselves, the part of our own identity that has been lost in our mobile and fast changing culture. Personally, I have difficulty coping with the quickness of change in technology. I can't even manage all the functional possibilities of the remote control for my VCR. I find myself confused many times by the sheer volume of information and number of choices available.

To minister to those with dementia we must be able to speak out of a common experience of what their confusion feels like. The challenge of caring with integrity is to allow our own aging and sometimes confused selves to serve as instruments of healing. (Isaiah 53:2-4)

CHAPTER 5

─────── ✿ ───────

THEOLOGICAL REFLECTION

"Can a mother forget the baby at her breast . . . ?
Though she may forget, I will not forget you."
(Isaiah 49:15)

People with dementia are a mystery to us. They can be a frightening mystery because we do not fully understand ourselves as human beings. Are we bodies with souls or souls having bodies or are these aspects of ourselves mysteriously intertwined in a unity? Is it possible to be a body without a soul? Does our value to God as human beings lessen when our intellect is impaired? Does the body remember even when the mind can't? These are some of the spiritual questions that arise when dementia is the issue.

Eugene Bianchi comments in his book, *Aging As A Spiritual Journey*, that within the mystery of aging there can emerge new possibilities and understandings for our own living.[1] We cannot explain this mystery, but we can respect it as having something to teach us about ourselves and God, and can trust God with it.

Dementia and aging raise the essential issues of life and its meaning when our options and choices are taken away. Spirituality is about confronting the boundaries of life and death. It involves grappling with hope and despair. The very stuff of the spiritual journey for those with dementia and for their caregivers is the experience of walking on the edge of mystery.

By caring for people with dementia in their full personhood, we grapple with fundamental questions about our own humanity, and about who and where God is in life. We are also forced to consider how we might reorganize our society in order to promote reverence for life in every form and state.

Theological reflection can offer some guidance in the spiritual care of those affected by dementia as we call upon the scriptures and celebrate God's presence in the lives of these special people. What is the theological foundation for caring and the mandate for loving those who lose their memories, who progressively forget their own lives, who forget their loves and who may even forget God?

Dementia is about chaos and confusion. Interestingly enough, the first scene of the scriptures is about drawing order and meaning out of chaos. (Genesis 1:2) Into this chaos God brought light. The light that God brings into the chaos of dementia may illuminate our attempts to learn what causes this condition biologically, to map its pattern of progress, and to discover medical resources to ease or eradicate it. Another light of God shining through the chaos might guide us in discovering how to live with people suffering from dementia, through developing coping skills that delay their need to enter a long term care facility.

Dementia is also about a wilderness experience, a central theological theme in the Hebrew and Christian scriptures. People with dementia are lost in their own confusion. They find themselves progressively entangled in the web of their own minds. Familiar landmarks of memory are absent. For both the Israelites, who wandered forty years in the desert, and for those who suffer from dementia, God continually leads and guards their lives by offering presence and care in tangible and concrete realities. God's guidance to those lost in the wilderness was not just spoken. Resources from nature (the pillar of fire and manna to eat) showed the way and made survival possible. As well, Israel was given sacred objects like the Ark of the Covenant and the Tent for Meetings. For those with dementia, spiritual care must be simple as well as tangible and concrete. Their promised land may be found in relationship with the caregiver, providing the security and love which are essential ingredients in survival.

Dementia is also about exile. In the sixth century B.C., the Israelites found themselves a defeated nation, exiled in Babylonia on the banks of the Chedar River. They witnessed the collapse of their most familiar symbolic systems. They lost their land, monarchy, temple, and independence. A deep sense of homelessness set in. The Babylonians asked them to sing a song to God. How could the Israelites do this when they felt God had abandoned and forsaken them? In their despair they said, "How can we sing the songs of the Lord while in a foreign land?" (Psalm 137:4) They had lost their sense of identity. They wondered if they could even survive without an identity. (Ezekiel 33:10) Like the person with dementia, the Jewish exiles were in an unknown land, surrounded by people alien to them, powerless, frightened, frustrated, angry and depressed. They longed for a time when they might see meaning in their existence, and evidence of God's love for them.

The prophets, however, declared that God's memory is everlasting. (Isaiah 49:14-15) Israel learned through this experience that she could survive by singing her old songs in a new way. The Israelites had to let go of their former ways of understanding God's presence and allow their symbols of faith to be transformed.

People with dementia have their own exile experience: the slow loss of independence, home and identity. Among the memories that do seem to linger, especially if there has been a church or faith background, are the old songs, hymns and symbols. These are important and lasting elements of identity. By singing the hymns, or even hearing them, they experience a profound way of being with their God that maintains their sense of connectedness and self esteem. For a person with dementia, seeing symbols and participating in the predictability of rituals are crucial to maintaining their spiritual identity.

Western culture emphasizes individuality and autonomy. Our philosophy of life is based on the factors of control, productivity and purposeful activity. We rely on our memory, our capacity to think things through. We expect to control our destiny and our bodily functions. The high value placed on control and autonomy springs from the Protestant work ethic, as developed throughout the Industrial Revolution and the Enlightenment. These values also fit well with the patriarchal mind set which underlies our patterns for allotting power in our social, cultural and economic systems.

Because of our western culture's penchant for control, waiting is understood as wasteful or even sinful. The condition of dementia abounds in waiting; thus, when people with dementia are unable to control their lives or do purposeful activity, they often feel useless.

Jesus described vividly in John 21:18 the plight of being older, helpless and no longer in control of one's life. He says, "I tell you the truth, when you were younger you dressed yourself and went where you wanted; but when you are old you will stretch out your hands, and someone else will dress you and lead you where you do not want to go." What a graphic picture of the elderly in the later stages of dementia!

This loss of control often results in anger and frustration. As we age, and especially when dementia is a factor, we need to recognize, accept and re-frame the realities of diminishment and waiting.

There is great mystery in the idea of being created in the image of God. One of the paradoxes outlined in the Christian scriptures is that Christ was the crucified God. Through this paradox, the divine image of the sufferer is affirmed. This is not promote suffering as a good thing which we should seek, but to recognize it as a reality of life which affects everyone, and in which we must still seek the Holy. For this reason we must value the times characterized by lack of purposeful activity as much as we value the active years. This enables us to see all ages and states, including waiting and dependence, as part of the created order. Seen in this light, the waiting figure can be one of extraordinary importance and remarkable dignity.

Violet is a resident who has taught me profound lessons concerning waiting and God. She is nearly 90 years old and has been waiting for death in the hospital for almost two years. Despite severe impairments, her central focus is scripture and prayer. While waiting for death, she still seeks life. Violet does not remember my name from visit to visit. She simply calls me "chaplain." She grumbles on occasion about physical discomforts, as anyone would, but I have never heard a word of complaint about her situation, the waiting state that characterizes her life. Her dedication to being a

Christian is not due to her great achievements, but it has a direct influence on who she is, and on the patience she displays in her waiting.

Can God be found within confusion? Is creativity possible in the midst of decline? Within diminishment there is the possibility of letting go of the things in which we have placed our confidence. In this release, we become more open to receive grace. To achieve this attitude one must accept the fact that there is never an ideal state in life, and believe that God is found in every facet of existence. Even diminishment can be approached creatively, aiming for closer relationships, the sharing of comfort, and the extending of oneself to others.

God does not spare us the little deaths, the diminishments of life, but rather transforms our weaknesses, according to St. Paul, into greater good. As Paul found ways to use his thorn in the flesh to understand more about God's love and faithfulness, diminishment can be an invitation to look for the Holy in human dependency. The condition of dementia causes us to enter more fully one of the paradoxes of life: growth through diminishment. It is valid for faith and hope that beneath, through and beyond the diminishments there is life-gaining power that will result in special good for humanity. Decaying seeds are a metaphor of this process. It is not the decay that brings the transformation, but the unrecognized, unbidden and hidden forces released in the process.[2]

In their own theological reflections, families I have interviewed whose loved ones are affected by dementia have said that they eventually discovered meaning for themselves even through their difficult experiences. Walter shares from his experience with his wife, who has progressed into a severe stage of Alzheimer's, that he has learned not to take life for granted, and has come to experience a peace that truly does surpass understanding. The close relative of an affected priest in residence says that she has come to perceive the need for understanding of the deterioration and has developed great appreciation for the ways in which people care beyond any sense of duty. Helen says that her experiences with her mother's dementia made her look carefully at what she believed about suffering and about a compassionate and loving God. Their life situations have propelled these caregivers to new depths of spiritual awareness.

Tielhard de Chardin speaks of two phases of diminishment that must be passed through in the process of life. He says that we must resist, with the help of medical intervention and research, the decline due to aging and disease. Nonetheless, there comes a point when the diminishment gains ascendancy. Then, and only then, does de Chardin speak of the diminishments' capacity to be transformed into resources for good. We release the old or let go to receive the new. When asked where creativity is found in the diminishments of the person affected by dementia, de Chardin suggests that the reality of life forces upon us a loss of self in our journey towards God.[3]

The self he speaks of is that Ego Self that resists the exposure of our Real Self. Paul Wilson, a member of the Christian Dementia Working Group in England, and a Methodist minister, poses a theological question: "If the ego is an inhibiting factor in our journey to God, are people with dementia more open to God (since dementia strips the ego of its power to mask real thoughts and feelings), and thus in a preferred position with the ego

replaced by a greater trust of others and of God?"[4]
Certainly our youthful prowess is furthered by an unin-
hibited cognitive ability that can even interfere with
transformation. In scripture, the apostle Paul speaks of
spiritual power being made known through weakness.
(II Cor. 12:10) When the ego is subdued, that which is
more divine assumes its place. The potential to become
more Christlike is created when the presumed power
and dominance of the ego are challenged by the weakness experienced through diminishment.

I have been privileged to observe that even in the
later stages of dementia, peoples' real selves are still on
a journey to God. Walter says of his wife that though
there is little (affective) response, there is, "a feeling,
somehow . . . a hearing, somehow . . . a knowing, somehow . . . that God is the Good Shepherd to her." The
close relative of the priest says that he remains in the
presence of God. His waking hours are filled with plans
for service, dispensing blessings and offering prayers.
These activities greatly help his present condition.
Helen relates that her mother is often in states of awe
and wonder when receiving the Eucharist.

In the book *Divine Milieu*, by Teilhard de Chardin,
passivity is said to comprise more than half of our life.
De Chardin says that the self is given to us far more
than it is formed by us. It is easier to accept the passivities of growth than to find God in the midst of the vast
and constant passivities of diminishment. Death is the
sum and consummation of our diminishments. It is the
critical point of union.[5]

Within the Christian scriptures we discover Jesus'
own struggle with passivity. In the midst of his passion
Jesus became passive. God's glory was revealed in the
Garden of Gethsemane when Jesus said, ". . I am he . . . ,"

(John 18:5) and gave up control of his destiny into the hands of his accusers. Although Jesus was handed over to wait upon and receive the decisions of others about his fate, and to become an object in their hands, God was no less God during this time of passivity than during Christ's active life.

In this image of Jesus there is hope, since passivity is such an inescapable reality for those who live in or with dementia. People may reflect the image of God no less when waiting passively than when working and achieving. Erosion of the ability to live actively does not diminish a person's humanity, even though our culture sees people with dementia as less than fully human.

Jesus was often asked to define himself and make clear his identity. He always did so metaphorically, with easily understood references to nature, creation and everyday life. For example, he said, " I am the true vine; you are the branches." (John 15:5) This unity that Jesus continually articulated was not simply an abstract thought but a description of his very being. The symbol of the vine describes the value of relationship for each person and thing in creation. In the moments when we sense our unity with all of the created order, we come to know who we are. Those with dementia are not segregated from the rest of the world or valued any less than God's other created beings. They are part of the created whole. Though the time may come when those with dementia no longer know who they are, they continue to be embraced in their full personhood within the community, and in the total circle of life, by those of us who know them and by the God who never forgets them.

When Pharaoh suggested that Moses take only the men into the wilderness to worship, we hear Moses respond, " We will go out with our young and our old, with our sons and daughters, and with our flocks and herds, because we are to celebrate a festival to the Lord." (Ex.10:9) The wholeness of society is dependent upon this wholeness across the age continuum.

Dementia is only one of the afflictions that can invade our lives, and it is certain to raise many questions. Is this disease a punishment? Why any disease at all? Certainly it is normal to be angry. Dementia is a killer. It destroys the mental powers of those we love through the destruction of their memories, the very things which make them unique. Whenever there is suffering, and when humankind's limited efforts are not enough to end it, the "why" question is asked. If God is all powerful, why does God not intervene to end our particular pain?

Perhaps one of the hidden gifts of dementia is the necessity it lays upon us to rethink our theology of an omnipotent God. Perhaps being God-like is not a matter of wielding power over creation so much as entering into the powerlessness of crucifixion. Perhaps we need to exchange our hopes that God will rescue us for a recognition that God accompanies us in our weaknesses and diminishments. Job asked similar questions as he sat on the ash heap covered with boils after losing all he possessed.

Might living in the later stages of dementia contribute to the completion of a person according to God's vision for him or her? Is this a possibility? Perhaps our perspective must change. Are we are being invited to channel our honest anger into more constructive responses? Can we become open to new insights? Maybe we are even asking the wrong questions. One resident's daughter eventually realized that dementia "just is."

So, what do we do with this state that "just is"? Coming to understand the life process in its reality is accepting the fact that no period in life is ideal. Our struggles and griefs mar our illusions of what life should be like. Grief resolution over time helps to bring an acceptance of the fact that this disease is not a personal attack of God on any one individual, but is part of the imperfection of creation as a whole.

Another question raised by cognitive impairment is how the mind, spirit and body are connected. Can we assert that our spirits remain when all else is gone? How much is one's faith understood as a product of the mind, the ability to understand God intellectually? We cannot fully comprehend God with our minds alone. We also need to actively cultivate an attitude of paying attention. Psalms 46:10 says, "Be still and know that I am God . . ." This concurs with my experience: I cannot know God by thinking alone, but but must actively pursue God's presence, nearness, love, creative energy and beauty in all that exists, including people who are severely cognitively impaired.

In seeking to discover God, two sources of revelation are creation and the incarnations of God. The first of these, creation, involves the experience of nature. Western theology has so emphasized the redemption theme, appealing primarily to the intellect through words, that God's revelation through nature has been a shadowy semi-acknowledged reality. Since time began, the earth has been looked upon as feminine, a womb from which all life came and the tomb to which we all return at death. Despite technology we are still in tune with its rhythms, but we have largely forgotten the patterns of movement of the sea, the enchantment of birds chirping, the delight of clear air. Despite our lack of awareness, the immensity of nature shouts out God's presence and creativity amongst us. Native Americans see God in everything. The Celtic tradition experienced the Holy powerfully through nature. The Jewish faith saw the natural world bearing witness to Yahweh God as well as valuing the Torah which orders human lives in God's way. (Psalm 19) If we allow ourselves to remember creation's powerful revelation, which transcends the cognitive, we can see God's touch even on those with dementia.

An intriguing study was done at the University of British Columbia concerning the effects of nature on people with dementia. An article in the Vancouver Sun, entitled "Gardens Have A Soothing Effect," published some of the findings of that study. It reported that violent incidents among Alzheimer's patients decreased dramatically when they had a garden in which to walk regularly. The UBC researchers couldn't explain or analyze nature's powerful influence, but speculated that contact with nature, even in an urban setting, is crucial for wholeness.[6]

Theological reflection brings some light to these surprising findings. In the Hebrew and Christian scriptures, creation culminates with the appearance of a man and a woman in a lush, wondrous garden. This suggests that from the beginning, spiritual wellness has been strongly connected with nature. To make certain that we get the point, we are told that humankind was formed from the humus or soil. The text (Gen. 2:15) asserts that Yahweh God put the earth-creature in the garden to tend and till it. The oldest creation stories from all cultures affirm the underlying unity of nature and humankind.

According to the Genesis story, Adam and Eve walked with God in the garden in the cool of the day. (Genesis 3:8) The venue of that meeting was as critical to communion with God as was the actual dialogue. Nature and humankind are intimately related, being created from the same materials of the universe and being dependent upon each other for continued existence. Even our most recent scientific theories of how the cosmos came into being affirm these understandings, for they tell us that all that exists has come from one source; we are all made of stardust. Many other biblical texts attest to the sacramentality of nature. In the book of Job we read the story which recounts the marvellous wonders of nature and creation: "Does the rain have a father? Who fathers the drops of dew? From whose womb comes the ice? Who gives birth to the frost from the heavens when the waters become hard as stone, when the surface of the deep is frozen?" (Job 38:28-30) Job replies, "My ears had heard of you but now my eyes have seen you." (Job 42:5) It is clear that Job's struggle was not what he thought it would be, a wrestling with God about the injustice of his sufferings. Instead Job looked into the natural world and knew God.

Such passages call us to see that nature is a bestower of grace, and may be a primary revelatory avenue through which God is experienced, even during the disease process of dementia. Our minds are closely connected to our bodily processes. A headache or tiredness for example, can frustrate our learning through the cognitive process. Research continues to demonstrate that the body has the capacity to regenerate and heal itself. Creativity, love, hope, and faith cause biochemical reactions which contribute to healing and a sense of wellbeing. At the most profound level, our spirits are created and recreated in terms of physical energies which are most intimately experienced through nature.

Many of my own observations concur with those of the UBC study. At our hymn sings, the favourite hymn by far is "In the Garden." It speaks of entering a beautiful, rose-filled garden alone, and of being joined by God, who walks with us through this garden. Even though they are not physically in a garden when this hymn is sung, the imaginations of those with mild to moderate dementia are often active enough to produce the same effects of calmness and peace that might result from actually being there. It seems that the imagery of the hymn has a healing appeal. As well, recreational therapists affirm that people with dementia have increased attentiveness and calmness in the plant care sessions. So, in various ways, people are soothed and strengthened by nature, and by contact with living, growing organisms.

A woman whose husband lives in the Dickensfield facility observed, after a small outdoor park was added, that the residents were hugging the trees, and said that the garden "gave them their dignity back."[7] One daughter commented that her mother, upon returning home from a hospital stay, literally skipped and jumped when she went into the garden. The peace that the person with dementia finds in a garden speaks very clearly of being at peace with the Creator.

Perhaps we who are cognitively intact are in large measure missing God's strong revelation through nature, as we asphalt our earth and as we depend so heavily on abstract concepts to understand God. The intellectually impaired are a challenge to our assumptions of cognitive superiority. They are indicators that we know less than we think, and that they know more than we have ever imagined. There is a great deal for those of us who are unimpaired to learn from people whom we have ignored because their mental processes are limited.

As advocates for those suffer from dementia, it behooves spiritual caregivers to promote contact with nature through open-spaced facilities which have gardens. Being in close contact with nature promotes a feeling of knowing where everyone fits in the larger scheme of life. It inspires the feeling of unity, and clearly brings joy. This is evidenced by behaviour changes: agitation and violence are replaced by peacefulness and calm. Perhaps we will also learn one day that treatment for violent criminals should be a matter of reconnecting them to the natural world instead of locking them away from virtually all contact with nature.

The word, "violence" comes from the Latin word *vis*, meaning "life force." Thomas Moore, in his book *Care of The Soul*, refers to violence as "the thrust of life making itself visible."[8] Our culture frequently chooses to be sedated to dullness and conformity, predictability and flatness. Perhaps there is a connection between violent outbursts and the need for surprise, the need to express passion, or the need for color in life, all of which are deeply spiritual needs. Perhaps violence is the drastic expression of a need for *vis*, the energy of life. The negative behaviors which coincide with cognitive impairment, such as agitation, screaming, wandering, aggression, violence, mood disturbances, hallucinations and inappropriate sexual display, may be more about natural needs frustrated in unnatural environments than about medical symptoms.

One of the most disturbing symptoms of

Alzheimer's Disease is that of wandering. Until recently, the accepted belief was that wandering was due to overstimulation. Straying residents have been given tranquillizers or other drugs to sedate them. Residential environments have been painted in soothing pastel colors in an attempt to discourage this troubling behavior. However, some exciting new evidence suggests that it may be an expression of the exact opposite: that people with dementia are more likely understimulated, and that their wandering may express a need for greater stimulation.

Some of the experiments suggesting this conclusion were conducted at the Edmonton General Hospital by a University of Alberta psychology masters student, Corinna Andiel, and reported in the Edmonton Journal on January 16, 1993. Corinna observed nine Alzheimer's patients, each for twenty minutes at a time over a two or three week period, and recorded their every movement. To avoid being noticed, she wore neutral colored clothing. Corinna observed that she rarely saw agitation or aggression but that, strikingly, residents were always running their hands over things and talking to each other.[9]

Andiel and Dr. Allen Dobbs, director of the Centre for Gerontology at the University of Alberta, agree that this activity is similar to the actions of children with attention deficit disorder, often called hyperactivity. The theory is that there is a basic level of stimulation that is appropriate and that, for some reason, it seems to take more stimulation to put the residents at the level of normal people. Something as busy as television is too complicated for many residents to understand. It is not enough that the resident be kept busy. "The stimulation must be meaningful to them," says Andiel. [10]

Looking at this activity from other than a medical model, we can wonder whether the purpose of wandering may be to find aspects of the lost self. Certainly in the Bible the wandering Israelites sought their lost identity, and the parallel to the dementia condition is obvious. It took Israel forty years (a lifetime) of wandering to move from their old identity as slaves to a new identity as a nation. Perhaps people with dementia are seeking meaningful stimulation that will help them find their identity. We need to take into consideration not only what they are feeling, but also what they are thinking. They seem to be trying to perpetuate the "I," the self. In the touching and talking that accompanies wandering they may be attempting to reclaim their connection with creation, which is the basic material of identity for the human being.

A very important element of a developing spirituality in anyone's life is attunement to the present moment. A spiritual directive from the New Testament says, ". . . now is the time of God's favour, now is the day of salvation." (II Cor. 6:2b). Getting bogged down in the past or fearing the future are temptations to which we can all fall victim. But there is another way to be. For people in advanced stages of Alzheimer's the past and the future cease to exist. There is only now. Each sufferer of dementia has a sense of reality based on his or her unique past experiences, relationships and personality. The conditions fluctuate, but even within the most severe cases of dementia it is possible for attentive people to reach in from time to time and for the person with dementia to reach out. When those with dementia attend to life, it may be because they have forgotten its complexity. Those of us that are cognitively intact allow the many demands of life to distract us from living in the moment; perhaps we need to be taught a similar simplicity.

Melody, although affected by advanced Alzheimer's Disease, notes my tiredness on some days or remarks when the colours of my clothing bring her pleasure. I have noted the sudden recognition of the beauty of a flower or the tune of a familiar hymn. I have seen childlike delight from tasting an ice cream cone after a hymn sing. I have noted that religion continues to be of value to those who have found it to be so in the past, even when the most severe stages of the disease are present. In Edna's case, she sought to speak and hold my hand when I read Psalm 23 to her one day, though she has never spoken a word on any other occasion.

An article in the November 3, 1992 issue of The Edmonton Journal was entitled "Dusk To Dawn." It is the story of the last days of a grandfather with Alzheimer's Disease. An accompanying photograph shows him holding his new grandson. The family speaks of his times of awakening, the lucid moments when their grandfather recognized them - the moments of "now." These moments were so precious to this family because he was really attentive.[11]

It is interesting that prayer and religion are often thought of as attending to the presence of God in the now.[12] Prayer has a very important function in the lives of those from a strong religious background. We must remember that prayer is not a scientific or medical technique, but a spiritual, mystical and intimate event. It is the expression of the spiritual relationship of the person with God. It is possible to see the results of prayer with someone who has mild to moderate Alzheimer's Disease and comment on it in the same way as one would describe the effects of pain killers, counselling or anti-depressants. Prayer calms, centers, focuses and gives peace. I have observed that it is as much the action of prayer as the specific words that makes a difference. The holding of hands and bowing of the head signal the movement into prayer. Jesus, in teaching his disciples how to pray, de-emphasized the number of words used when praying and even chastised those who made a display of their ability to pray with many words.

For those with dementia, the power of prayer is found in its freedom to express the reality of the feelings of the moment. Whether life is being experienced as good or bad at the moment, expression of feeling at the time of its happening is important. It is a way to unload, to be connected with creation and the Creator. Prayer is also a way of opening to intimacy that can exceed person-to-person levels of communication, especially for those with dementia. No one knows or understands them as well as God, making prayer especially therapeutic.

The essence of prayer for those with dementia is not about actually obtaining a desired result; it is the experience of expressing one's desires, as a child would ask a parent for attention or favours. Affection and comfort flow from simply being close to the parent while asking. The act of prayer as spending time with God makes the relationship with God more intimate.

The book, *From Image to Likeness*, describes four pillars or wellsprings from which our lives flow. These pillars, which are the ways we experience God, are sensing, thinking, feeling and intuiting.[13] To see, to hear, to smell, to taste, and to touch are all gifts of God. Augustine thought that it is God we ultimately see with our physical senses. We often think of the soul as being in the brain, but it may be more true to human experience to locate the soul in every part of the body. Thomas Aquinas spoke of God being in every living thing. God is ultimately in music, in nature, in beauty and even in that which we perceive as ugly. Those with dementia seem to allow reality to touch them through all their senses, at unpredictable moments. Such experiences provide energy for them in the form of stimulation, pain or pleasure.

Is memory the recollection of events in life, or is true memory participation in, not merely nostalgia about, life? I would suggest that dementia is a forgetting of one's private memory, but even into the last stages of dementia, real participation in life happens primarily through the senses. A communal memory can make meaning possible. The wonder produced when those with dementia attend to God speaks of their capacity for the Divine. Perhaps our part as people who are less cognitively impaired is to witness to and celebrate this capacity.

One of the major fears of those with dementia is that the essence of their self will be taken away and their personal dignity destroyed. The goal of spiritual care is to maximize individuality and independence within the community where the gifts and lives of those with dementia would be cherished. This care must value the individual's personal autonomy and dignity. To communicate this, the caregiver must make an effort to learn about past interests, names of grandchildren, hobbies and other pertinent information. Recognition of each individual's right to respect and dignity must be foundational in the caring center's mission statement. Verbal and tactile messages of concern, support and love reinforce dignity. These qualities maintain contact with the humanness of the person.

Thomas O'Connor, in his article "Ministry Without a Future," (Journal of Pastoral Care, Spring 1992) writes that when he visited a long term care facility, he pondered what gift he would want to give them. He decided that he would want them to know that God thinks their lives have been worthwhile and that God loves them and will take care of them. In this regard he realized that providence was their major spiritual concern.[14] Paul Pruyser, in his book *The Minister As Diagnostician*, outlines eight religious concerns, of which providence is one. Providence can be defined as the intention of the Divine towards oneself.[15] O'Connor says that those who are affected must trust that providence looks beyond this thing called senile dementia. Though the time may come when they no longer remember names, they have sufficient emotional resources to develop feelings of security and trust in their caregivers, through whom they can experience God's providence.[16]

In the story of the valley of the dry bones, from the book of Ezekiel, the movement from death to life rests upon the action of the Holy Spirit. Israel was given an inner and deeper gift: God created a new identity for her. The Spirit of God is able to replace what is lost with something new. Each person with dementia is still on his or her faith journey. We should not underestimate the power of the Holy Spirit. An example of this is Agnes, a resident of Anglican background. Agnes could recognize shapes, but could not remember her own name. She had a mantra that she repeated constantly. "Thank you, Jesus. Thank you, Jesus. Thank you, Jesus." She asked Jesus to lead her to her room. After prayer she was silent for a moment and then said

"Amen." Her deeply ingrained faith in Jesus maintained her identity for her.

Worship cues or faith memory cues, the strongest of which is probably the Eucharist, can be instrumental in how the Holy Spirit maintains the identity of each person. Helen says of her mother that even in the severe stages of Alzheimer's Disease, Pearl has times when she seems to be experiencing awe. She is also able to participate appropriately in rituals, such as the taking of bread and wine. She responds to the priest in his vestments and seems to sense the do's and don'ts of the church.

For the ancient Hebrew, the ultimate loss was to be forgotten. One of the greatest issues in my grief for the gradual loss of Grammie McCloskey was that she had forgotten me. Since our mothers, fathers and grandparents mold our first images of God, perhaps there is an archetypal fear released in us when a parent or grandparent is affected by dementia, the fear that God will ultimately forget us.

One man ponders about his mother in the book *Winter Grace,* by Kathleen Fischer. "My mother used to be God's good friend. She prayed to God three times a day as a devout Jew. She cared for her mentally ill sister and was a faithful visitor to the sick. God has become a stranger to her as have all her good friends. She mentions God's name from time to time as if wondering what became of him. God seems as hard for her to locate these days as a hair pin. "[17]

The passage from Psalm 88 reminds us that God's remembrance of us is not dependent on our own limited abilities or capacities for private memory. A final word comes from a daughter: "One thing I used to wonder about was my mother's relationship with God.

If she was so confused that she had forgotten Him, would He still remember her? Then one day the answer came very clearly into my mind. My mother had forgotten about me, but she was still my mother, and I knew and loved her. In the same way, the Lord knows who are His. That was it! God knows, and as long as God knows, it does not make the slightest difference whether we know or not ourselves."

CHAPTER 6

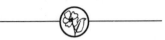

SPIRITUAL ASSESSMENT

Spiritual assessment is desirable in order to determine how the spiritual wellbeing of the individual affects their overall ability to cope, and to determine what avenues of ministry best meet the specific spiritual needs of each person.

Spiritual assessment is not an end in itself. Rather it is the first step in the clinical pastoral task. Assessment leads to an impression, a diagnosis of the spiritual issues that are pertinent to the care of the person affected by dementia. Determination of individual spiritual issues then leads to the development, implementation and evaluation of a plan of care.

The assessment is a series of judgements, based on such things as whether the resident is open to care, how they feel about the facility, their emotional state and the spiritual history, background and operational theology of the resident. Based on a consistently applied model, spiritual assessment must clearly identify the issues that are relevant to the spiritual care of the resident.

In this context, "spiritual" is defined as that aspect of the human experience grounded in certain universal needs and yearnings pertaining to one's meaning in life; realizing a sense of self, both apart from and in relation to a group, and maintaining a sense of union with that group which may be seen as transcending self.[1]

Spiritual sensitivity is not always synonymous with religious practice and so assessing spiritual life needs may be very complicated. Even for the cognitively intact, spiritual assessment is an exercise in paradox. This is pointedly illustrated by Jesus' saying, on the one hand, "By their fruits you will recognize them . . ." (Matt. 7:16) and on the other, "Many will say on that day, 'Lord, Lord, did we not prophesy in your name?' . . . then I will tell them plainly, 'I never knew You'." (Matt. 7:22-23) Spirituality   itself is a complex and somewhat vague concept. Add to this the vagueness of dementia and the problem is compounded. A person with advanced Alzheimer's Disease cannot produce the kind of "spiritual fruit" generally thought of as evidence of a healthy spirituality. Further, such people eventually forget even their religious foundations and cannot remember to pray or to communicate in any observable way with God.

To create programs and activities that enhance the spiritual functioning and fulfilment of the individual, we need a tool which allows us to look at spirituality as an identifiable variable. The form of the assessment tool must reflect the realities and limitations of the health care facility and the individual's stage of dementia. It must also be user-friendly, such as a check list of items to consider when assessing spirituality, or a listing of considerations and issues.

Each person has a unique spiritual style in the way he or she seeks, finds, creates and uses symbols of faith. The concepts of Greg Stoddard and Jean Burns-Haney outlined in their paper, "Developing An Integrated Approach to Spiritual Assessment: One Department's Experience," encompass the spectrum of considerations that require assessment for a person affected by dementia. Paul Pruyser's categories inform the model further from the perspective of traditional theological terminology:[2]

Assessment Area:
Pruyser's Diagnostic Categories

Concept of God . . . . .Awareness of the Holy

Subjective meaning of illness . . . .Sense of grace

Approach to hope . . . . .Faith relation

Support system . . . . .Communion

Figure 3

The following diagram illustrates how the assessment model and themes affect each other: [3]

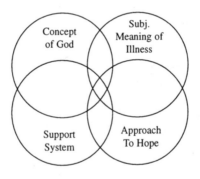

Figure 4

By "Holy" I mean the human experience of the wholly Other, an overwhelming experience of that perceived to be wholly outside of one's ordinary experience.

Meaning-making is possible in the mild stages of dementia and includes one's ability to trust, to give and receive acceptance, and to feel appropriate responsibility.

The factor that differentiates resignation from acceptance is the ability to maintain hope. What is the content of the resident's hope and how is he or she relating to that content? If hope is tied to a cure, it can devalue participation in present relationships and prevent the individual from looking towards the future realistically. It can also be used to avoid experiencing the present moment. Hope is a function of that in which one puts one's trust (faith) and a sense of assurance that such trusting will serve a constructive purpose. Despair happens when choice is lost and life is no longer a matter of trust but of necessity. The challenge of hope in chronic and life threatening illnesses is the re-framing of one's expectations in the light of the new circumstances so that choices remain.

The support systems that are assessed include: family and other significant people, organizations, churches or other faith communities and the staff of the facility. The task of the chaplain is to assess how well the elements of the support system work.

The support system and the resident may be in conflict in a number of ways. The resident may need to talk about his or her situation while the family may find it too frightening. The condition may cause people from his or her church to feel hesitant to visit. On the positive side, the support system may provide consistency in love and attention. As well, if conflicts arise within the system, a chaplain is usually able to act as mediator. Communion encompasses the full range of issues that bind together or estrange.

While the spiritual assessment model provides a lens to view the spiritual state of the individual, the method of its application insures that the model is effective and consistently applied.

Use of the model is limited to other than crisis situations. It is to be conducted only with the permission of the resident (or, if the resident is unable to speak for herself or himself, the resident's family).

The chaplain needs to discuss the results of the assessment with the resident and a plan of care must be agreed upon by the resident or family. The best approach is the less intrusive method of conducting a standard non-directive pastoral interview and using the model to later reflect on the content. This assessment utilizes the four themes shown in Figure 4.

Prologue Note to the
Spiritual Assessment Model:

When the dementia is still in the earlier or less severe stages, the following spiritual assessment questions could be posed directly to the resident. However, if it has been determined that the dementia is moderate to severe, these questions are best directed to family and/or friends, upon their willingness to respond.

Section II contains questions regarding those who have been the resident's primary caregivers immediately prior to their arrival at the long-term care residence.

SPIRITUAL ASSESSMENT (A MODEL)

NAME OF RESIDENT:

FORMER ADDRESS:

DATE OF BIRTH:

DATE OF ASSESSMENT:

CLOSEST RELATIVE:

SECTION 1
ASSESSMENT OF RESIDENT

GENERAL INFORMATION:

1. Describe the resident's stage of dementia:
   a) mild
   b) moderate
   c) advanced

2. From the history of the resident, what were or are their interests and hobbies?

3. Does the resident have physical disabilities that affect living now?
   a) hearing
   b) sight
   c) walking
   d) other (specify)

CONCEPT OF GOD:

4. Does this resident know a sense of reverence and awe?

   If yes: a) How is it expressed?

   b) How is the Holy experienced?

5. Is God important to this person at his/her present stage of life?

    If no: Was God ever important?

6. How would the resident describe God?
   a) loving
   b) just
   c) judgmental
   d) remote
   e) other (specify)

7. How would the resident describe what God does for him or her?
   a) loves
   b) cares
   c) helps him or her keep on living
   d) judges sins
   e) not much help
   f) nothing
   g) other (specify)

8. What do you observe in the resident's behavior?
   a) tears
   b) wringing of hands
   c) wandering
   d) aggressiveness
   e) gentleness
   f) anxiety
   g) grief
   h) anger
   i) other (specify)

9. Does the resident appreciate:
   a) scripture reading
   b) poetry reading
   c) formal / informal prayer
   d) other (specify)

10. What faith symbols and rituals are important to the resident?
    a) the sacraments
    b) crucifix
    c) rosary devotions
    d) sweetgrass ceremony
    e) other (specify)

11. What faith-related services seem important to the resident?
    a) chapel services
    b) mass
    c) communion
    d) visits by clergy or church members
    e) other (specify)

12. What holiday occasions are important to the resident?

13. What type of music does the resident like?

SUBJECTIVE MEANING OF ILLNESS:

14. What gives meaning to the resident's life?
    a) God
    b) spouse / family
    c) friends
    d) being alive
    e) life achievements
    f) activities
    g) other (specify)

15. What has previously been most important for the resident in life?
    a) God
    b) spouse / family
    c) friends
    d) career / achievements
    e) activities
    f) other (specify)

16. To whom does this person turn when most afraid?
    a) God / Jesus
    b) Allah (or other diety - if so, specify)
    c) spouse / family
    d) friends
    e) clergy person
    f) church
    g) support groups
    h) doctor
    i) professionals in the institution
    j) no one
    k) others (specify)

17. What does he or she do when afraid?
    a) watch television
    b) walk or pace
    c) find someone to talk to
    d) pray
    e) meditate
    f) other (specify)

18. What bothers the resident about living here?
    a) the feeling that their life is over
    b) the feeling that he or she is not ready to die yet
    c) wondering who is responsible for her or him
    d) feeling like a burden to everyone

e) feeling abandoned by loved ones
f) lack of privacy
g) loneliness
h) having nobody to talk or socialize with
i) fear of strangers
j) being unable to sleep / awaken on their own timetable
k) their health
l) the food
m) other (specify)

APPROACH TO HOPE:

19. Where does the resident find hope?
    a) God
    b) spouse / family
    c) friends
    d) nature
    e) professional care
    f) other (specify)

20. Does he or she still have choices, or perceive that choices are still available to her or him?

SUPPORT SYSTEM:

21. Does the resident find their family and friends supportive?

    If yes, in what ways?

22. Does the resident actively belong to a church, faith community or support community?

    If yes, what is its name?

23. What can the institution do to make the resident feel at home spiritually here?

Note re: Question 24 (below) -
This question is to be answered only if the respondent is a caregiver, i.e., someone other than the resident:

24. What nonverbal communication do you find most effective with your loved one?
   a) touch
   b) music
   c) play activities
   d) aroma
   e) colour
   f) humour
   g) other (specify)

SECTION II
ASSESSMENT OF PRIMARY CAREGIVERS

NAME OF PRIMARY CAREGIVER(S): _____

ADDRESS: _____

POSTAL CODE: _____ PHONE: _____

RELATIONSHIP TO RESIDENT: _____

DATE OF ASSESSMENT: _____

25. Do the family and friends of the resident seem open and receptive to the idea of their loved one receiving pastoral visitation and/or interventions?

   If yes, what support can be offered?

26. Does the family seem open to receiving pastoral support in their on-going task of caregiving?

Once an assessment tool is in place, the caregiver will review it regularly and make any needed revisions to enhance the effectiveness of the individual care plan. The primary means of evaluating the care plan is through a quality assurance process. This process monitors the resident's refusal and/or acceptance of pastoral care visitations. It also includes a subjective evaluation as to the improvement or decline of quality of life of the resident and notes the input of staff and family as to the support offered.

The spiritual assessment tool would best be implemented and evaluated in an interdisciplinary team setting under the leadership of the chaplain.

Spiritual assessment, unlike a medical diagnosis, must intentionally look at the whole person in a way that is positive and affirming. Such assessment will take into account the physical, emotional, psychological and spiritual dimensions as well as the support offered by family, friends and community. The degree of cognitive impairment and the capacity for involvement in various aspects of life, which would seem peripheral to a medical and physiological assessment, will be important aspects of a spiritual assessment.

CHAPTER 7

ISSUES OF GRIEF AND LOSS

Grief and loss are profoundly important issues for those who suffer from dementia, as well as for their family and friends. Grieving the losses through a duration of up to 20 years is extremely demanding.

Those affected by dementia not only must come to terms with the usual spiritual issues, such as the acceptance of being older and the likelihood of the eventual loss of home, possessions, and community, but they have the added grief of anticipating the loss of their abilities to comprehend, remember, and make good choices. Grief is especially common in persons suffering the early symptoms of dementia. People do not become progressively impaired without having an emotional reaction.

Counselling those with declining cognitive ability is a fairly recent venture. It was commonly believed that intervention was too difficult to attempt, and that even if it were possible, its effectiveness would be shortlived. In 1988, Labarge, Rosenman, Leavitt and Cristiani undertook a pilot study, the findings of which were reported in the *Journal of Neuro Rehabilitation*.[1] There were twenty-two participants in the study. The age of the participants ranged from 68 to 84 years, with the mean age being 74.04 years. The study was composed of twelve men and ten women. All the candidates were assessed as having mild Alzheimer's type dementia and being free of clinical depression.[2]

In the initial stages of the disease, individuals possess more than fragments of comprehension, although what they understand is masked by aphasia and short term memory loss. Qualitative results from this study indicated that under the category called "inherent strengths" were the personality traits such as flexibility, the ability to see oneself humorously, and the patience to handle uncomfortable situations. The researchers discovered that the essence of many facets of a healthy structured personality remained, even as cognition eroded. Under the category of "maintenance of the mastery of life skills," these abilities were appreciated anew as other abilities faded. The study found that a positive self concept was preserved longer for those who had a life history of accomplishment and felt secure in their competence, such as an airline pilot or the mother who had reared children. Family and friends, as well as philosophical tenets and spiritual bases were found to be important in positive coping.[3]

The most important cognitive strategies that this study discovered were the pep talks that people gave themselves and their attitudinal changes, such as not being embarrassed anymore when they couldn't remember names. They learned to wait for people to introduce themselves with the understanding that since they couldn't change what was happening, they might as well choose to calm down and make the best of it.

The spiritual task in grief work with those affected by dementia is enormous and requires a great deal of patience from the caregiver. Depression (in the person with dementia or in the caregiver) is a human response to loss, and is very common. Depression becomes harmful when something interferes with the giving up process and the depression is prolonged. In my encounters with residents struggling with their grief, I have observed that a lack of family support and presence and a lack of spiritual background are enormous inhibitors to recovery from depression. Depressed sufferers from dementia rehearse over and over the litany of reasons why they no longer want to live. At the time of one visit I had with such a person, the nurse commented that she had never seen the resident smile; she just wanted to die. In my visit, I merely showed interest in her and listened. This brought her some happiness and she began to see life differently.

Those in the mild stages of dementia can experience a whole range of emotions and share their pain with others in seeking support. They anticipate losses in abilities. Listening to their concerns can help them work through their feelings of sadness. Diminished memory makes this a more difficult process in the moderate stages, but it can be done, albeit at a less verbal or even nonverbal level. Life long personality traits are likely to be enhanced by the condition of dementia. For example, rigid people become more rigid. In consequence, those whose religious belief system has emphasized judgment may need particular reassurance that they did not merit this disease by being sinful.

In her cognitively intact years, my grandmother McCloskey had a quiet, unassuming and pleasant personality. This did not change in the later stages of her life. Her caregivers in the nursing home where she eventually lived commented that she never complained and was most patient.

The spiritual caregiver should not rush in with pat answers or try to make everything better. Pointing out previous sources of strength is helpful. Reading a familiar verse of scripture can provide a sense of security in an insecure world. For many, prayer is a key element offering hope as a way to overcome loneliness. To pray with another person is also an affirmation that someone cares for them.

Those suffering from dementia need to be recognized and respected as people made in the image of God, and as having a valid need to grieve. Fran, who was in the earlier stages of dementia, told me that her tears could fill an ocean. These are the times when those affected by dementia feel intense anger at God because of their fear that God has forgotten them. They identify with the psalmist, who said, " How long, O Lord? Will you forget me forever ? . . ." (Psalm 13:1a)

Often it is comforting for the resident who has a Christian background to hear the story of Jesus on the cross. They relate to Christ's expression of feeling forsaken, and his anguish at God's absence. For those whose verbal skills have vanished, just to see and hold the symbol of the cross is sometimes enough to bring this sense of comfort.

Grief and loss create a more complex issue for the confused than for those whose cognition is intact, because their sense of time is altered. Linear time gradually ceases to exist for them. They enter a state that one would almost call an eternal time. There is no logical succession of events; everything happens in the moment, in a perpetual present time. An anonymous writer has created an image of life. For those of us who are cognitively intact, time is like a stream of water in which we float with the current. For someone with Alzheimer's Disease, time is frozen into individual snowflakes that touch the skin and melt.

Martha's husband died last fall. The arrival of a trustee on the unit with some legal papers created in her the belief that her husband had just died that day, although he had actually died a month earlier. Time for her had frozen into one moment. My intervention that day was to listen to her grief and validate her feelings all over again, as if it were happening that very day, just as I had on the day he actually died. Because the one with dementia can experience a loss over and over again as if it were constantly happening in the present moment, the caregiver, like the person with dementia, must respond to an altered sense of time.

An understanding of grief resolution is very important for the caregivers of those affected by dementia. Listening to the feelings of the confused person is no less important than listening to the feelings of a cognitively intact person who is experiencing a loss. Failure to recognize and validate the grief negates the person. Conversely, listening to the expression of emotion affirms the grieving individual's personhood. This task of listening is likely to require repetition because the reason for grief is not remembered as having been in the past, but can be experienced afresh at any time.

Roles change in the family structure as the disease progresses. This can be a great source of sadness for the caregiver but may be even more painful for the person affected by dementia, especially in the earlier stages. Role reversal means a parent or spouse becomes as dependent as a young child. The losses experienced need to be mourned. It is very difficult to accept that even though they are physically alive and present, the one who used to listen, nurture, and give advice and affection is no longer able to do so. The parent grieves that they are now like the child. Many emotions and tensions may arise when this role reversal manifests itself. Helen, a caring daughter, noted very clearly during her interview that role reversal was her greatest challenge in caring for her mother since the onset of dementia.

Dementia is a disease of separation. Lily was a very good example of this. She spoke of her great sadness in not being able to go home where there was no one able to look after her. She lamented constantly her inability to work anymore, as her work had supported her sense of self worth. She missed her father, whom she thought was still alive. She missed her home in Prince Edward Island. Acknowledgement of such losses was central in my ministry with her. Before she died, Lily expressed gratitude that I had listened to her.

One task of dementia-related grief work is to emphasize familiar patterns and experiences that continue, such as relationships and various aspects of nature (seasons, sunrises and sunsets, etc.) Life's rhythms are another important continuity. Most standard songs approximate our heart rate, so music that matches our body's systems can enhance our sense of security and wellbeing. Because consistency, rhythms and patterns are so important to people with dementia, grief work with them requires consistency in caregiving, ongoing presence and patient listening.

Hope allows us to see things in a new way by throwing something novel into the equation. In grief work the primary task of the caregiver is to instill hope. The Bible tells of just such an incident in Luke chapter 24. Two men were walking together on the road to Emmaus. Their mood was one of heaviness and hopelessness; they had been crushed by the death of their leader and friend. With downcast faces they poured out their story to a stranger who joined them. Their hope had been that Jesus would have set Israel free. They were so despondent that they did not even recognize Jesus (the stranger) nor could they imagine the possibility of a different result. Jesus, through a discussion of the scriptures, tried to tell them that all had been fulfilled, but not in the way they had expected. Hope lives in the matrix of faith and is open ended. It provides a wider perspective to our limited ways of viewing things. By caring about the needs of the stranger and offering to share their food and shelter, hope came alive through the breaking of the bread.

The hope of the person grieving the progressive disease of dementia is that they should not to be abandoned. Presence conveys the incarnation of the Holy. This keeps alive their hope that they will be comforted in times of confusion, grief, loneliness and fear.

For the caregivers and the loved one affected by dementia hope can be enhanced by helping them connect their human story to the greater divine story. This is what happened on the Emmaus road when Jesus spoke from the pertinent passages of scripture, and explained his (and consequently their) place in it. We need to liberate human wounds from isolation. When this happens, linear time, *chronos*, is transformed into eternal time, *kairos*. Strangely enough, even for those of us who are cognitively intact, our most profound and blessed moments have been the the ones imbued with that sense of eternal time.

The family caregivers have a double burden to bear. The day-to-day strain of providing constant care is compounded by their need to deal with the grief they and their loved one are experiencing. It is helpful to identify the stage of the disease through which the loved one is passing. Similar to the Catholic observance called the Stations of the Cross, it helps us to say "yes" to where we are now. There is great comfort to be found in this type of acceptance.

Caregivers therefore must be proactive rather than reactive to the progress of the disease. They may need to also re-grieve each loss or change in the person. They should be encouraged to become familiar with the grieving process and to validate their own feelings and experiences, which are a part of the process of greater self understanding and spiritual growth.

A chaplain colleague, Rita Sandmaier, has proposed three stages of grief resolution in the condition of Alzheimer's Disease. The first stage is separation. There is separation of the loved one from the usual way of life and from the community. The second stage is marginality. The cognitively impaired person no longer has a voice or way of participating meaningfully in the community. The third stage is reintegration. This brings a renewed understanding of the purpose of life with the understanding of the changed identity of the loved one.

Initially, diminished ability to remember causes insecurity and anxiety. The person feels more and more vulnerable, nervous and agitated. At this stage there can be fits of anger. In the more advanced stages the person enters a state of calmness and indifference. One of the graces of dementia is that the memory loss prevents them from being aware, especially in the later stages, of the seriousness of their condition.

Earlier, I suggested that perhaps what those affected with dementia fear most is the loss of the essence of the self and of their personal dignity. At the Alzheimer's Day Center in Columbia, South Carolina, staff, families and volunteers are called the A-Team. The Center was founded in the belief that it is possible to care for persons suffering from dementia in a community-based setting, where individuality and independence are maximized. It was designed with a structured, stimulating environment, geared to positive, nonthreatening and life enhancing opportunities that bring out the person's remaining abilities and skills. The Center's cornerstone of care is the commitment to consider people in their totality, in their full personhood. They are not patients defined by their disease. They are viewed in the broader sense of their past experience and within the context of community. Experience is valued over textbook approaches. A relative of a woman at this Center is deeply moved with relief and gratitude when she sees her loved one maintaining a perception of her own dignity. The beloved resident wants to wear her nice dress, always with stockings and good shoes. She pretends she can still read. She has lost almost everything, but not her dignity.[4]

One woman, speaking of a loved one affected by Alzheimer's Disease, says that the condition was hard to accept because the cognitive changes were in such minute increments, and there was no particular physical change, such as their might have been after an operation. Accepting this phase of dementia is a slow process. Those whom I have interviewed and those about whom I have read have coped best with the grief when they accepted help in the midst of their helplessness.

As a chaplain in a long term facility where dementia abounds, I see patterns of response both in the victims and in their caregivers. As Martha O. Adams says in her book, *Alzheimer's Disease*, "I have witnessed where the foundation of religious faith begins to emerge. For those who have a strong faith to sustain them in such a trial, the going is not easier but different. Those with a faith background ask the same questions, suffer the confusion of no answers and agonize with doubts, but the difference is the assurance that we are not alone. Meditation and prayer are oases of refreshment in days of grief." These are what Oakes calls rhythms of reliance; acknowledging one's difficulties and weaknesses, and then giving up and soaking in the Holy for the strength to go on.5

Judith is a resident who, in dealing with the losses in her life, is comforted and strengthened by these rhythms of reliance. Often when I encounter her she is sitting in her wheel chair at a table with her head in her hands. She seems so despondent and lonely. The offer to pray or read scripture with her invariably brings a clear, positive response. After this refreshing oasis she seems energized, and unfailingly expresses her gratitude.

The losses and grief due to dementia in those who are also experiencing the usual restrictions of old age demand our special attention and care. What is the price of their dignity and emotional well-being? It is one which can be paid by generous caregivers, in the currencies of attentiveness, validation and love.

CHAPTER 8

THE ROLE OF REMINISCENCE

The long-observed inclination of the elderly to live in the past, once a cliché, is now understood to be a critical element of spiritual wellbeing.[1] Although the onset of dementia inhibits storytelling to some extent, nonetheless making connections to the past begins a process of healing.

At the most basic level, reminiscence provides pleasure and increases self esteem. It offers contact with others and diminishes the sense of isolation. More importantly, reminiscence satisfies the need for a sense of continuity, a bridge to reality, a sharing of their world, a climate of appreciation and a time of celebration. In the Christian sense, it means resurrection or seeing things anew. Activating the faith memory helps maintain a sense of identity in God's family.

Reminiscence is universal. A review of literature on developmental tasks suggests there is an important search for a narrative line in old age.[2] The person experiences being a self through the telling of the life story. Our lives are made up of events, occasions (pleasant and unpleasant), memories, successes and failures. Memories of these experiences through which we have lived are embedded deeply within us. Rarely do we slow down enough to step back and review our memories, but there comes a time when we must do so.

Because dementia affects the remembering and

telling of stories, the caregiver often hears only fragments. A person affected by dementia may even feel that there is no story to tell. Encouragement may often be needed from the spiritual caregiver to initiate reminiscence. Residents' stories may need to be enhanced, focused or given momentum. Such is the case with Chester. He tells bits and pieces from his days as a coal miner and frequently downplays the importance of his life. During my visits with Chester I encourage the telling of his story and assist him to link its parts.

Lily was one resident who revelled in telling me about her younger years on Prince Edward Island and the events of her adult life. Recalling her job as an accountant affirmed her sense of meaning in her life. She remembered that teaching had not been her first love, so she had taken the risk of leaving that career to pursue work that she found fulfilling. She told this part of her story with great satisfaction because of the courage she had displayed. It gave her hope to talk about going back to PEI. Her relationship with her father was central to her other relationships. She had been married twice, but had no children of her own. This memory caused her great pain.

Jean is another example of someone very attached to the telling of her story. She had taken a trip to the Holy Land, to which she referred after each hymn in our regular worship times. This journey to the Holy Land seemed to be a time when her experience of Jesus was at its most concrete and meaningful, because she had walked where he had walked and stood at the place of his crucifixion and resurrection. Her memories of the Holy Land trip served to maintain her Christian faith and identity.

The position taken by Robert Butler in the 1960's

was that reminiscence can arouse unresolved intrapsychic conflicts with the reality of approaching death. Review can bring one to wisdom, courage or serenity. It can also lead to depression and despair for those whose choices have lacked deep integrity. This is now recognized as a limited view of reminiscence. A more current understanding of this activity is that reminiscence maintains and restores the sense of self of the individual.[3]

In the earlier stages of dementia reminiscence is an especially important activity. Reminiscing can also be "future oriented," serving as part of our preparation for ending the life story with consistency. As listeners we are mirrors for the person affected by dementia, validating their stories. This raises their self esteem, calms and reassures. Since dementia can cause distorted self narratives, it is the task of the listener to offer reinterpretations of the person's life story, with genuineness and thoughtfulness, in ways that enhance self esteem, and sustain a sense of self by uplifting with hope.[4]

Reminiscing reminds us that each of us is "an original." One of the amazing lessons I have learned as a chaplain is that the telling of our life story allows us to feel loved and unique. The cognitively impaired are more isolated than most people because of their inability to express themselves coherently. For the person with moderate to advanced dementia, memories of the distant past are often more available to recall than those of the recent past or the present. Creative methods are needed to establish avenues for expression. I have found it helpful to use storytelling cues, such as pictures of family, friends and significant places or events. Stories then come more easily. As well, the physical environment should enhance and not inhibit the storytelling. Sharing most easily takes place in quiet, private living areas of the facility.

The listener must display a non-judgmental attitude of acceptance. People who tell their stories to find meaning in their life can see God's faithfulness reflected by someone who cares enough to listen attentively. The caregiver (who may have heard the same story many times) will have to exercise great patience, drawing upon their moral and spiritual commitment, to listen yet again to what is Holy to the storyteller. The caregiver must have no particular agenda, but be ready to go where the storyteller leads and be oriented to that reality. There is a quality to such listening that is incarnational, embodying the loving respect of God.

The caregiver will look deeply into the eyes of the other, observing every facial expression and nuance. If a verbal response seems desirable, he or she should speak quietly, slowly, calmly and gently. This requires being focused and undistracted. Because of the decreased attention span of a person with dementia, it is better to have frequent, short episodes of story-telling (no longer than fifteen minutes), rather than infrequent but longer sessions.

For one woman in more advanced stages of dementia at the General Hospital, a very common statement is, "My name is Rita Parker" (her birth name). I always have the sense, because she says this so emphatically, that she is striving to assert her identity. In the article, "A Biblical Basis For Telling Stories," author Mary Lashley speaks of meeting a ninety-four year old woman called Esther. At first she was anxious about how to reach a mind so distressed and confused. Listening over a period of time, Mary discovered Esther to be a deeply religious person; raised in the Roman

Catholic church, she valued receiving the sacraments and prayed daily. During many of their visits, Mary and Esther prayed. Despite her memory loss and sensory deficits, Esther's prayers were deeply ingrained in her memory. Though she stumbled at times, a little prompting helped her recollect a line or a verse. Her prayers also invited Mary to participate in the storytelling, sharing family and life experiences that centered on her own religious faith. Once in the midst of a fervent prayer, Esther abruptly stopped, looked at Mary and remarked, " Jesus has been good to me." Then suddenly her countenance changed as though a new idea had come to her. With certainty and self assurance she exclaimed, "But do you know something? I have been good to Jesus. Yes. I have been very good to Jesus." Esther was saying that she was faithful to her God in word and deed.[5] Esther's self-esteem was tied to her faith, and it was through the sharing of her unique story that she made this important discovery about herself.

A poem called "Endings," by Lynn Kozma (from the book, *When I Am An Old Woman I Will Wear Purple*) is a poignant picture of reminiscence in the moderate to later stages of dementia:[6]

ENDINGS

Frail as porcelain
she sits, unmoving
except for bone thin hands
mending with care
forgotten clothes
which are not there -
threading unseen needles,

moistening fingertips
from parchment lips,
knotting the thread
carefully.
There - once more finished -
smoothing the wrinkles away,
softly laying it by,
slipping back
to the early May
of her life
as easily as breathing.
My planet - earth;
hers - a distant star.
Impossible to travel that far.

by Lynn Kozma

In my many chaplaincy visits I have discovered that not only do those affected by dementia maintain their sense of identity through reminiscence, but they also appear to be energized by the activity. Jean is an example. The recollection of her parents' singing engagements and recording sessions caused her countenance to light up; even her posture became more erect with excitement and joy. Nell is another woman who smiles continuously as she tells her story, and seems to have more vitality after the reminiscence. I have found that the listener can enhance these story-telling sessions by asking open-ended questions that lead the speaker to recall more details. It is highly fulfilling when both speaker and listener can enjoy the process, celebrating the story together.

CHAPTER 9

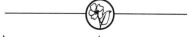

ALTERNATE APPROACHES
TO SPIRITUAL CARE

I t is no exaggeration to say that our western society is highly cerebral. We lay so much emphasis on the verbal that inarticulateness is billed as inferior by a society enamoured of speech. Artists tend to be poor; musicians fare much better; authors are considered most successful. Matthew Fox says in his book, *Original Blessing*, that a theology of the word of God is being killed by the word of God. Fox suggests that the *dahbar* (creative energy) or word of God is more right brain (having to do with affection, love and play) than it is left brain (cerebral and verbal), and yet we expect the verbal to communicate more than it is able.[1] Almost seventy percent of all communication in our world is nonverbal. Therefore it seems a safe assumption that contact with wisdom means going beyond words.

A common misunderstanding about the resident with dementia is that if the affected person cannot converse verbally, no communication is possible. This is the same mistaken assumption that is sometimes made about young children before they are able to speak. At least with children we attempt to communicate constantly with facial expressions, holding, touching and playing.

Ministry to those affected by dementia needs to become increasingly nonverbal as the disease progresses. This was the case with Howard, a resident with whom I found verbal communication to be of little effect, yet his sensual perception remained highly efficient. Touch, music and color brought life to his eyes. Because he experienced these ways of expressing care, he also made attempts to interact nonverbally.

Possibly the most profound of the varied means of nonverbal communication is what I call "presence," the simple act of being with another person. Presence is powerful, yet is often overlooked or forgotten because it is not a cerebral activity. We often fail to recognize the power of presence until someone is suddenly absent from our lives. It is an article of faith in pastoral care literature and in the experience of caregivers that presence communicates the love of God. I have had innumerable caregiving experiences in which a profound sense of presence was expressed in silence. When I began to visit pastorally, I had to learn to appreciate the power of presence. I held the mistaken belief that nothing was happening when there was silence. I attribute my initial discomfort with silence to my over-reliance on verbal communication. As I became more aware of the power of presence and silence, the passage "Be still and know that I am God" (Psalm 46:10) came alive for me, and perhaps so did God.

MUSIC

"I hear you singing.
The music you bring is a thread
weaving the frailties,
bridging the gap that distances us.
All with gentle persistence
Constant like the sea, a part of you alive in me . . ."[2]

Lois J. McCloskey, from *The Silent Heart Sings*

Throughout history, music has shown itself to be a healing force. The philosophies of sacred sound are found in most ancient religious traditions. Quantum physicists agree with the mystics that the universe is vibrating and pulsating. The standard rhythm in most songs closely matches the human heart beat. Paul Nordoff and Clive Robbins, two pioneers in music therapy have stated: "Music is a universal language. It has been called a nonverbal language."[3] We are rhythmic beings. It is supposed that our sense of security and wellbeing is linked to our sense of rhythmic pulse. Our earliest experiences of rhythm and pulse, essential to our very survival, are the womb's constant echo of the maternal heartbeat.

Miriam suffers from severe dementia and is also very deaf. She is one of about 30 people who attend the unit hymn sings on Monday mornings. The piano there has quite a penetrating tone, and she sits quite near. She often taps the rhythm on the arm of her chair. She participates in no other way, but she expresses her pleasure in the moment by joining in the rhythm, to which her physical being can still respond.

The Greeks used music to strengthen character as well as to eliminate disease. Illness was understood as disharmony and music personified and restored harmony. In the Bible, I Samuel 16 tells of King Saul, who was frequently overtaken with a spiritual malady. When David played soothing melodies on the lyre, Saul's spirits improved dramatically. In dealing with a condition that affects the brain and the intellect, it is exciting to realize that there is readily at hand an avenue of communication that can extend to the farthest reaches of the human soul.

When music is used for healing, music therapist

Helen Bonny Lindquist defines the process as "a systematic application of music to bring about changes in spiritual, physical and emotional wellbeing. It is a functional, as well as an entertaining medium."[4] Catherine, a woman of 82, suffered from terminal cancer and mild dementia. A Catholic, she had found great comfort in God throughout her life. Music soothed her, diverting attention from her physical pain. Her frequent comment was "You have no idea how much better I feel." Just before she died she was overcome with gratitude for the beauty of music and she said to me, "God really loves us."

Music therapy is especially helpful in ministry with those suffering from dementia, for it communicates with the healthier parts of the whole person, creating alertness and stimulating memory, emotions, motor skills, and psychological responses. Joan Butterfield Whitcomb, in her article "Thanks for The Memory," says she believes that neural pathology is circumvented, at least during the time of the musical interaction.[5] Her statement is based on observation of over two hundred Alzheimer's residents in adult day care centers, a field in which she worked for more than a decade.

Long before I became a chaplain, I was profoundly impressed by a healing moment which occurred through the use of music. At that time I worked for a home care agency called Comcare. One of my assignments was to help a man, Richard, with his household tasks after he had incurred back injuries. His wife Suzanne was afflicted with Alzheimer's Disease and eventually was placed in a long term care facility.

I had heard about music therapy, and since I also knew Suzanne through my role as a lay pastoral hospital visitor, I thought I would try an experiment of my own. I asked Richard what Suzanne's favorite musical piece had been in her younger years. He told me it was "Greensleeves." I found the piece at the public library and when I next visited her I played it on the stereo.

The response was amazing, even phenomenal. A huge smile came across an otherwise expressionless countenance. Her eyes had a sparkle in them. She literally lit up. Her emotion was visible everywhere and was obviously one of joy and happiness. It was if she had returned from a distant land. I have never since doubted the power of music to improve the quality of life for severely cognitively impaired people. In part, this experience was my inspiration to use music extensively as a chaplain.

Music is essentially an emotional event. In the mild to moderate stages, the cognitively impaired have ready awareness of their feelings. Even those in more advanced stages of impairment experience feelings, although less predictably. Music mobilizes unimagined resources, offering the scope to explore intangible issues and the freedom to venture from cognitive understandings into the realm of the emotions.

The experience of music is something that is difficult to capture in words. Perhaps there would be no need for music if it were possible to communicate everything verbally. The depth and breadth of music is akin to the depth and breadth of emotional expression. It is a safe place to work through emotional issues. Irene, a 64 year old woman, asked for loud, quickly paced hymns when she verbally expressed anger, and when feeling sad she requested quieter hymns.

How do we know that emotional issues are being worked through rather than simply felt? I have noted less fear and anxiety, increased alertness, and greater openness to relationship in those residents with whom I have used music extensively. These observations lead me to believe that there is more going on than simply an experience of emotion. Behaviour is being affected. Music has the potential to express diverse themes simultaneously, as do the emotions. We can possess neither music nor our emotions as objects, but we can experience both of them in the present, moment by moment. The human psyche is composed of conflicting information, meaning and feelings, all seeking expression and satisfaction. Hope, anger, grief and regret may all be present. The music therapist may not be able to specify the particular issues with which the listener is dealing, because that person can't easily verbalize the journey. In fact, the accepted meaning of the music may be quite different from that perceived by the person with dementia. But I have observed that when the music provided has been meaningful in their past, particular feelings that are unique to that person are often expressed. The experience and expression of such feelings often leads to a sense of satisfaction, which may be conveyed through a smile, the seeking of eye contact with the therapist or a calmer, more relaxed demeanor.

I would describe music as "the soul's language." It is not surprising that music is one of the best resources available for promoting spiritual wellness. A holistic approach to personhood is superior to a mechanistic one, which sees the person in terms of a collection of component parts, each of which can be treated separately from any other. Because our spirituality is addressed as much emotionally as intellectually, music becomes a powerful element of healing and integration, bringing wholeness to the disoriented and distressed.

For two years, I have co-led the weekly hymn sing in the facility where I work. Up to thirty people now attend these musical gatherings which began with approximately twelve. I also lead hymn sings in the rehabilitative units, where cognitive impairment is frequently accompanied by other health problems.

I have observed that not only do the residents seem more alert and relaxed after these sessions, suggesting that the experience contributes to a higher quality of life for them, but the direct care staff seem happier and more relaxed as well. That this can be attributed to the music and not other factors is supported by the staff's appreciative comments, by their singing or humming of the songs after the music sessions, and by their frequent requests for particular tunes. Positively influenced staff members show more patience towards the residents' behavioral disturbances and are more attentive to their needs. In short, music diminishes stress in the entire facility.

The well known journalist Bill Moyers has published a book, *Healing and the Mind*, which explores this exciting new understanding of the connection between the mind and spirit. Another resource is Tom Harpur's *The Uncommon Touch*. Both acknowledge the power of the senses to enhance life.

The article, "Ministry With the Confused Elderly" also observes, with utter amazement, the improvement that is often evident in residents when the minister conducts hymn sings in public worship. A group that seems completely out of touch with the world becomes a worshipping community and needs no more direction than an unaffected gathering.[6]

These effects are particularly observable with Norma at my Monday morning hymn sing. Norma's level of cognitive functioning is very low. Although she cannot remember my name, the glimmer in her eyes speaks of recognition at some level. She cannot maintain a conversation of even the shortest duration, but she loves to sing and can sing many lines to most hymns. Norma's medical chart indicates that she has no memory capacities, yet she hums the melody when she isn't singing the words, and does so quite beautifully. She directs with her hands in spite of the fact that they are crippled with contractures. The music seems to prompt these rhythmic movements of her arms and hands. She has a wide vocal range that most would envy. After the sessions she is much more energized and alert, and appears less tense. It seems as though her body remembers, through music, what her mind can no longer recall or hold. When Norma is in an irritable mood, just singing a few words of a hymn takes her out of the mood immediately and she breaks into song. The transition from agitation and irritableness to happiness is not gradual, but instantaneous. It changes the spirit within her. Her entire demeanor brightens considerably and she sits up straighter. In the past, Norma played the piano, painted, hooked rugs and read. As these abilities slipped away, her capacity to enjoy music remained.

Music therapy also relieves boredom. People with severe dementia sit silently on the unit for countless accumulated hours. Music provides a stimulating way to fill this emptiness with life. Joan Butterfield Whitcomb states, "If one can imagine oneself with little or no short term memory, with no sense of the environment and no familiar points of reference, one can only imagine what a relief it must be to fill one's mind with pleasing and familiar sounds."[7] Music helps transcend these limitations of daily existence. It expands life in the present moment by sweeping the resident into a reliving of precious moments from the past. We have all spent time as children imagining ourselves in many different places, doing a variety of things that were not possible in reality, but which stimulated our imaginations and gave us a unique kind of liberty. This creative and deliberate pretense is known as "transcendent voyaging." Music is one of the means through which the experience can be accessed.

It is of interest that Dr. Nahama Glynn published an article entitled "The Music Therapy Assessment Tool," in which she states, "No specific reference has been found in the literature regarding the use of music as a therapeutic modality with Alzheimer's patients."[8] This statement is refuted by the research of Clair and Berstein (1990) whose study of music therapy for severely regressed persons with Alzheimer's type dementia revealed that despite ongoing physical, social and cognitive decline, these persons can continue to function in structured music group experience.[9]

Millard and Smith (1989) found that therapeutic singing groups increased designated social and physical behaviors and that selected music activities even increased cognitive performance as measured by the Folstein Dementia Rating Scale.[10] Prickett and Moore (1991) found in their study that people with Alzheimer's-type dementia demonstrated greater accuracy in tasks requiring recall of words to familiar songs versus tasks requiring recall of spoken words alone.[11] This again supports my observation that music-related activities improve quality of life.

Nurses are able to provide opportunities for music on occasion. But in times of economic restraint and financial cut-backs, such as we are experiencing now, they have little or no time for activities with the residents beyond the performance of basic nursing tasks. This means that the responsibility for using music to enhance the wellbeing of Alzheimer's residents often falls to the spiritual caregiver.

The performance and enjoyment of music has always been a communal activity. This makes it especially valuable in long term care settings where isolation from family and friends is often an unhappy reality.

Active group singing can help form emotional bonds, because it makes participants feel good about those with whom they share in producing these happy sounds. Residents not only listen passively, but as their abilities permit, take part in making the music. Community is built as residents gather for the hymn sings. We acknowledge our loss as a community when a resident dies. I have heard residents humming on the way back to their units, knowing them to have been silent when they came. They always interact with much greater sociability after a hymn sing than before the event.

Sharing music is one of the most effective activities I do in my work as a minister. But obtaining the best response from the cognitively impaired requires the use of hymns and songs with which they were familiar in the past. Many of these people grew up through childhood and into their earlier adult years singing around the piano at church or on other social occasions. It is clear that hymns in particular, relax, calm and uplift people with dementia. This is even true for the staff and visitors who share in the music. Christian symbols evoke reverence and awe, and this response appears to be deeper when music is part of the experience.

When I began the hymn sing sessions I used tape recorded music, believing that the residents would be more responsive to this passive approach. Quite frankly I doubted that the music I could make myself would have as positive an effect as a professionally produced product. Later, I started to use live music by playing the piano in response to direct requests. It didn't take long to notice the difference. More people attended and the responses were much more enthusiastic when the music was created by someone in the same room. It seems that the form of the presentation makes a significant difference. This experience was confirmed later in an article by Lucanne Magill Bailey, "The Effects of Live Music Versus Tape-Recorded Music On Hospitalized Cancer Patients," which stated that the presence of the human being, body and voice, as an originator of the sounds provided a stronger stimulus. The live music has an energizing effect between the source and the listener.[12] By leading the singing, and putting my whole self and energy into it, I found a way to release the residents to do the same.

Meaningful words combined with a comforting familiar melody seem to be stronger than words alone. Repetition pays great dividends during music therapy with those who are cognitively impaired. It heightens their self esteem and consequently their spirituality to be able to join in a chorus with energy and assurance.

The hymn sings provide repetition, familiarity, routine, predictability and positive reinforcement, all of which are vitally important, life-strengthening elements. Familiar selections (especially the old hymns) make an unfamiliar and threatening environment feel safer and more secure, thus opening up the possibility for interaction and communication. Two residents,

Irena and Mildred, both answered "Yes" when I asked them if they enjoyed the hymn sing. This is extraordinary, as both are severely affected by dementia and speak very little. Irena does speak some Ukrainian to her family, but I have never heard Mildred speak a word of English in the two years I have known her. Her hands are severely contractured and she sits very straight in her wheel chair with her tongue rotating in her mouth constantly. She always looks to be in great distress. One woman whose symptoms are less severe said one day, following a hymn sing, "You just can't replace these old hymns." Indeed, they are unique and irreplaceable for the task of making the unfamiliar familiar.

Music can also be used creatively as a bridge for people. When we sing "He's Got the Whole World in His Hands," I insert the names of the residents into the song. Their reaction is profound. They become much more attentive and alert. Music therapist Lois J. McCloskey suggests that residents are enriched by "singing about the people they have touched, those they have loved and contributions they have made throughout their lives."[13]

Music creates a meaningful connection with the present; a sense of wellbeing is restored for a precious interval of time. The words and tunes fade soon after the event, but the positive effect lingers and can be built upon. Music therapy can be part of a holistic approach to facilitating the person's optimal level of functioning. Quite simply, music produces joy.

Music also supports reminiscence. This reality was revealed to me by Jean, who was moderately affected by dementia. She would weep as she sang because she was reminded of her singing family, especially her parents. Her short term memory decreased dramatically over her time in the hospital, but long term memory remained intact. I suggested to her that in the moments when she shed tears called forth by singing, memories of her parents were being vividly recalled. Recognizing the truth of this brought great comfort to Jean.

The older hymns that are familiar to the elderly from childhood are the most desired forms of music at our facility. Helen Bonny Lindquist has done research which leads to a similar conclusion. Her article, "Music and Healing," states, "It is concluded that in serious illness there is created a right brain propensity for reception of meaningful stimuli. Great music that has lived through time is more readily accepted on physical and intuitive levels."[14]

Lois J. McCloskey, in "The Silent Heart Sings," tells of a program she developed called "Reprise," in which music is combined with reminiscence and life review. In her experience, music facilitates word retrieval and long term memory. She focuses on recalling a memory and then sharing the reminiscence. It is important for the caregiver to listen and accept these feelings without judgment.[15]

Music is tremendously powerful. Fequency, intensity, intervals, rhythm, tone and tempo transmit potent nonverbal messages and touch the human emotions beyond cerebral control. At my hymn sings, I deliberately shape the session by building a rhythm into the structure of the event, moving from slow to fast paced pieces and ending with a quiet series of hymns. I have discovered that exaggerated mistakes in piano playing draw additional attention and laughter. As well, I make a point of planning sessions to reflect the rhythm of the seasons with special attention to holidays, thus providing constancy amidst experiences of disorientation and loss. Music is also a highly effective, non-pharmacological intervention in pain control. Research has shown that it engages affective, cognitive and sensory mechanisms, by changing the perception of pain, altering the mood, enhancing control, using prior skills and promoting relaxation.[16]

R.R. Parse in her theory of "becoming," (described in the article "Consider Karaoke") speaks of meaning, rhythm and transcendence as the three themes linked to health. Parse says that human beings live their present, past and future simultaneously. The present holds memories of the past and ideas for the future. Thus the meaning of present experiences includes what is, what was and what will be all at once.[17] Residents often speak of the past, returning to childhood memories of church and family life. Jean recognizes how much closer she feels to her parents since the hymn sings began. She has become much more contented and at peace, as memories of beloved people and past events representing her identity have emerged from her memory.

Through everything from a subtle nodding of the head to toe-tapping or the tapping of a hand on the wheelchair, residents reveal the impact of music. Some cry; the melodies draw them to express their feelings.

When conventional language fails, the thoughts and feelings of people with dementia are often unrecognized or ignored. Music moves beyond external language and affirms the emotions, providing an outlet for inarticulate feelings and a way of participating in community with God and with others.

PLAY

Can God be experienced through play? I have observed that the ego, which shrinks as a result of dementia, prefers literalness in activities, while the soul seems to love play. As stated in Thomas Moore's book, *Soulmates*, the preoccupations and concerns of everyday life are not exactly the same things that nourish the soul.[18] The human species is unique in its capacity to remain playful into adulthood. Sadly, we have not fully appreciated the power of play to help us know God or to develop into spiritually healthy individuals. Matthew Fox suggests that our patriarchal society has poisoned play.[19] Yet God is our divine playmate who calls out the child in all of us so that we can share godly delights and enter God's kingdom (Matt.18:3). In wisdom literature, the Song of Songs compares the play of God to the playfulness of lovers. Western thought and experience have been dominated by redemption theology, which views humans and creation as essentially sinful, in need of correction and forgiveness. This theology tends to perceive solemnity as a virtue. A creation-centered theology, on the other hand, celebrates God with joy, seeing all of life as essentially good, a blessing from the hand of God.

At the very heart of play is rhythm. Religious growth encompasses chanting, singing, laughter, and other rituals and activities that involve rhythm. All these events are open to the participation of people affected by cognitive impairment. In their situation of mental and spiritual pain, playfulness can soothe and unburden the spirit. Yet play suffers if it becomes too intentional. It has to be spontaneous and free and so requires activation of the creative playfulness inherent in the spiritual caregiver.

Unit 8B is the locked cognitive support unit at the Edmonton General Hospital. One winter's day, tables were placed together and the recreational therapists brought in a pail of snow. Spontaneously, residents began to make snow balls, scooting them them across the tables at each other. The unit chaplain observed that spirits were amazingly lifted by this childlike activity. For that time they were enjoying life, and in the process, enjoying God who is life for us and in us. Similarly, the simple activities of throwing around a large beach ball or painting pictures for fun have brought far greater pleasure to the residents than might have been anticipated. The twinkle in their eyes is a beam of clear, joyous light shining out from their souls.

Residents also enjoy playing with sand, water and wood pieces. One of the great gifts of childhood is the pre-schooler's ability to become lost in simple play activities. Those with dementia seem able, at times, to become immersed in a similar, unselfconscious and highly satisfying type of play.

One day I brought a piece of kinetic art to the unit. It was a silver circle that rocked rhythmically back and forth. Within the circle was a smaller circle with three balls mounted on a black base. Continuous movement was made possible by a battery. Though the circle was perfectly steady in its pace of rocking, the three inner balls on the smaller circle spun chaotically within the larger circle. Lily was fascinated by the toy, and deeply puzzled by it's continuous motion, but she still laughed at the random spinning of the inner balls within the larger circle. In the environment of a long term facility, which has so much predictability built into its schedule, Lily was delighted by surprise. Certainly predictability is necessary in this environment to prevent anxiety for the residents, but Lily yearned for some gentle novelty. My own spirituality has often been enlivened by the God of surprise; perhaps, for those few moments, Lily's spirit was playfully surprised too.

Dolls are another important object of play and a wonderful resource to fulfil the need for a mother or mothering symbol. In the article, "To Find A Soul, " the authors told of 90 year old Dinah, a woman in the terminal stage of Alzheimer's, who was unable to walk, talk, smile or swallow. She lay in a fetal position, her face flat and expressionless. Her only family was a sister, Sheila. One day Sheila brought in a doll, and a remarkable change came over Dinah. As Sheila placed the doll in front of her, Dinah's face lit up and she said quite clearly, "Oh, darling, look at the baby." The nurses watched in amazement as her clawlike fingers reached out gently. Making cooing sounds, and smiling all the while, Dinah nuzzled the doll, cuddled and caressed it. She has since become more vocal and even though much of what she says is incomprehensible, she sounds happy and content.[20] When Miriam, one of our residents at the General Hospital, was given a doll to hold, she awakened to a happy awareness of her ability to give love.

The recreational therapists on Unit 8B have noted that more women than men seem to be attracted to playing with the dolls and teddy bears. However, in the article "To Find A Soul," the authors tell of Duncan, a former engineer, who was not interested in magnetic blocks or large puzzles, but delighted in a brown teddy bear. Then there was Rupert, who preferred a slice of cheese and a cold beer to teddy bears or blocks. Generally, however, the article concurs with our therapists' observation that dolls provide comfort and companionship for most residents.[21]

An area for future research is the effectiveness of clowning, miming and liturgical dance as additional alternative approaches to providing spiritual care. Such activities might open the doors for afflicted people to express their identities through physical movement.

An activity suggested by one of our recreational therapists that soon became a part of the weekly hymn sing was eating ice cream. From the very beginning, the residents were as eager as children to have a cone. Wilma, a woman who attends the hymn sing on Monday mornings, shows no particular response to the music. But she sits up, eyes wide open, and eagerly reaches out for her creamy treat. Her childlike enjoyment and delight in this simple pleasure is the epitome of play. Playfulness is Godlike; in their enjoyment of ice cream, residents resemble the God who looked at creation and saw (surely with great delight!) that it was good.

HUMOUR

Humour has been referred to by a humour therapist as playing with your pain. In *Prayers For A Planetary Pilgrim*, Edward Hayes uses the image of a tightrope walker. The way of life is narrow and no one would venture without a balance bar. Balance brings inner peace. We cannot maintain balance if we are tense and rigid. We need to be flexible, able to sway from side to side. Humour provides the balance bar.[22]

At a recent public forum held to raise funds for the new proposed Alzheimer's care centre in Edmonton, Suzanne's husband Richard stated that there is nothing funny about life when taking care of a person with this disease. After a period of time though, he said, we can look back and see the humour in things that were said or done. The key is to find the incongruities of life in the situation. To be able to laugh in the darkest of gloom is a paradox that can lead us to the Holy.

Through humour and play we are able to forget our everyday problems and move into a new frame of time, a type of timelessness which is a taste of the eternal. Timeless moments of eternity are ecstatic experiences located in the heart of our experience of God.

Among the severely affected, the ability to be humourous seems to come from within their personality type. There are many residents who never smile anymore. Others laugh regularly. Grace chuckles and giggles after almost every attempt at speaking, then peers intently to see if I will join her in her amusement. Perhaps her frequent laughter is an attempt to gain acceptance and approval. Humour seems to be her pathway to acceptance and unconditional love; this is one way to experience God. Olivia is another resident, moderately to severely affected, who often responds to people and situations with humour. One of her common words is "honey." Once, when Olivia wanted the attention of a chaplain colleague, she called, more and more loudly, "Honey . . . Honey . . . HONEY!" When the chaplain responded by coming to her, Olivia grabbed her by her skirt and said, loudly and with a huge smile, "HONEY!" I find Olivia's way of seeking attention quite endearing. Recently I met her on my way to another unit and stopped to chat. She had a beautiful purple flower tucked into her tightly wound bun. When I commented on its beauty and on how nice she looked, she grinned in a way that only Olivia can, and said, "Yeah!!!"

A chaplain colleague has shared her experience with Ellen, a woman in the severe stage of dementia. At one point, Ellen became very ill and a priest was called to administer the sacrament of the sick. Ellen did recover from her illness and the next week my colleague remarked how very well she looked. Ellen responded, "I don't know about that!" Responses that evoke laughter are not uncommon. Ellen seemed to understand at some level that the chaplain was referring to her recovery from the illness, even if she was not exactly ready to agree that she looked well.

Martha O. Adams, in *Alzheimer's Disease*, notes that a sense of humour can help us through even the worst of times. She confirmed that her father's sense of humour had not only remained intact, but continued to develop. One Saturday morning her father was in high spirits when she spoke to him on the phone. "I want you to know I woke up this morning with a woman named Marilyn next to me," he said. "You did?" Martha quipped. "You mean Marilyn Monroe? Wow! How did that feel?" "Well," he replied, "it was quite remarkable. She even had on one of your mother's nightgowns." "Really," Martha remarked, "Now that's amazing." "No," he said, "The amazing thing is . . . they look so much alike."[23]

Adams tells another humourous story about a time when she was visiting her parents, both of whom were experiencing dementia to some extent. Her father started toward the bathroom and her mother followed. He turned to her with a twinkle in his eye and pronounced with dignity, "I'm going in to shake the dew off the lily." As he gently closed the door behind him, Martha's mother looked at her daughter and said, "Nothing can get him down . . . where DID he go?" Adams told her mother where her father had gone. Softly, so he would not hear, her mother inquired, "Do you suppose a man like him ever gets married?" "You've been married to him for fifty three years," the daughter smiled. "I have?" questioned the mother. "Then I guess I don't need to worry." Martha also noted that annoying questions can be turned around or difficult situations diffused by seeing the humour in them.[24]

There are a thousand instances in a long term care facility where the caregiver can find humour, laughing not at the residents, but with them, acknowledging our human solidarity in the funny things that make up life. One Monday morning when I asked a woman in quite advanced stages of Alzheimer's to our weekly hymn sing I received a very different response than usual. That particular day she retorted quickly at my invitation, "Mind your own business," and then she chuckled. She was teasing me and she enjoyed it.

Lily was another resident who enjoyed a humourous moment. She was one person who was particularly interested in my wardrobe. Although I have occasionally worn a longer leather skirt, my usual skirt length is just above the knee. Lily always found it humourous to tell me that my skirts were too short. While scolding me, she would sheepishly try to hide her smile with her hand; her eyes would dart here and there, pretending that she feared I might get upset with her. Of course I was never was upset by her joking. In fact, I found it endearing. The shared laughter brought us closer because it allowed us to be ourselves.

During chapel services, residents often make comments which bring a smile to the face, perhaps because they are so close to what we think or would like to express, but are too inhibited to say. One such occasion was a service near Christmas. We were singing, "glory to the newborn King," and at every chorus one of the residents would sing clearly above the rest, "glory to the newborn Queen." Here was a true feminist! The content or length of chapel services have also prompted such comments as, "What's that got to do with it?" or "It's about time!" Such quips and comments reinforce my belief that humour expressed and shared is a deeply human response, which persists and brings joy in spite of Alzheimer's.

NATURE

Even those of us who are cognitively intact have had our souls shrivelled, our imaginations confused and our psychic energies dissipated by our alienation and isolation from nature. It is a vitally important, foundational human need to have contact with the natural world.

One person describes visiting a nursing home that was bright and sunny, and filled with various animals. Colorful parakeets and canaries sang. Kittens chased each other over and under chairs, and around and through potted plants, tumbling over each other along the way. They jumped into laps and purred and rubbed their feline faces against human ones. The residents were made happy by these animals.

Mildred's absorbing interest is cats. She has cat pictures of every kind literally papering her room. She has stuffed cats and cat toys. On her last birthday, I gave her a cat my daughter and I had made from wound yarn. Of course, she had owned cats throughout most of her life. In this long term care facility, it remained the one

thing which was life-giving to her. Recreational therapists and volunteers bring in cats and dogs regularly
for the residents to stroke and enjoy. For Mildred, who
suffers not only from dementia, but from several other
major debilitating problems, cats bring pure joy in a
world otherwise dominated by suffering. Pets remind
us that God is present even in our pain. They affirm
that we are loved, and indeed, lovable.

One evening recently I went with Helen to visit her
mother, Pearl. As the three of us strolled through the
facility, we came upon a caged yellow budgie. Pearl
stopped abruptly, captivated by the chirping of the
bird, and then looked over to see my reaction. It was if
she wanted to share the joy of the moment.

Another place God is recognized profoundly is
within babies. One day a staff member on maternity
leave brought her newborn for the residents to see.
Many of them were overwhelmed by the experience.
They reached out and gently touched the baby's tiny
limbs, or softly stroked the downy hair. Their smiles
and luminous eyes were impossible to miss.

Gardens and other experiences of the natural world
can be a way for the person with dementia to experience God. We have inherited from traditional Christian
theology a tendency to value dominance and disem-
bodied spirituality, and to mistrust nature as a pathway
to God. Nature is not merely a secondary place for
quiet and peace. The images of nature seep into the
souls of those affected by dementia and burst forth with
unexpected energy. Exciting recent additions to the
resource base are the "environmental" tapes that use
nature sounds either on their own or in combination
with music.

These needs for intimate contact with nature have

implications in the present use and future planning of health care facilities. As facilities stand now, resident's rooms and common areas could be enhanced with living, growing plants. Walks in the park could provide hands-on contact with the natural world. It is also critical that future projects be developed with parks and gardens in and around them. The goal should be to make available to the resident as many opportunities as possible for direct contact with nature.

SYMBOLS, RITUALS, SCRIPTURE AND PRAYER

"Then Mary took about a pint of pure nard, an expensive perfume; she poured it on Jesus' feet and wiped his feet with her hair. And the house was filled with the fragrance of the perfume." (John 12:3)

Clergy and other caregivers may feel overwhelmed by the spiritual needs of people with dementia. Conversely, they might neglect those needs altogether, thinking that since these people are already confused, spiritual ministry with them is irrelevant. This is a consequence of the belief that the intellect is the main and perhaps only way of learning. Caregivers may not understand the use or impact of such ministry tools as nonverbal communication or physical symbols.

Spirituality means much more than belonging to an organized religion. Among other things, spirituality reflects the wellbeing of the whole person. Many current approaches to physical healing emphasize the need for mind and spirit to be enlisted in helping the body to heal. The opposite is also true, that the body can be enlisted to help heal and maintain the spirit. The sense of permeable boundaries between the body and the spirit also characterizes our relationship with all of creation. We are realizing that we cannot precisely define where the body stops and where external nature begins. Books such as Bill Moyer's *Healing and the Mind* and Tom Harpur's *The Uncommon Touch* are recent publications that emphasize this holistic thinking.

All of our relationships, whether with others or with God, are mediated through our bodies. Our senses and feelings bring the world to us. Our minds and spirits are affected by how we relate physically to the world. God is experienced by us through the material, the medium by which we connect to the world. Jesus is quoted as saying that what we do to the least valued of our companions in creation is what we do to him. (Matthew 25:31-46)

In ministry to those affected with dementia, as with any other form of suffering, hope is essential. To share hope we must use the best possible means of communication. This is the same attitude with which we minister to the terminally ill, seeking access to the hoping self, that dimension of the person where hope resides.

Research is being done by Dr. Ronna Jevne and others at the University of Alberta, through the Hope Foundation of Alberta. During a seminar at the General Hospital, Jevne reported that when terminally ill patients were asked where they placed their hope, their answers were, "Taking care of my plants," or "The smell of cinnamon buns," or "Looking at a mountain and lake." All their responses were very simple and concrete. The circumstances of hope were very clear and tangible to these patients. Hope is found in the discovery of our permeable boundaries and body experiences, and its foundation is our connection with the rest of creation. Jevne wonders whether hope is primitive, like sound, sight, and smell. Her intuition is telling her that hope might be found more in the realm of appetite and passion, than in the realm of the cognitive. In essence, Jevne postulates that hope cannot be separated from the physical condition. Perhaps hope is a renewal of our primordial intimacy with the natural world. Experiencing God in nature (as discussed earlier in this chapter) and finding the Holy mediated through our bodies would support the suggestion that spiritual elements, such as hope, can be conveyed through the concrete, natural world.

That which is Holy in life must be recognized, even if in a limited fashion. Faith symbols and religious rituals are not perceived totally with the intellect. They reach people at an emotional level, and thus can evoke a response that connects the person with God, life, the energies of the universe and the rest of humankind.

When a priest administered the sacrament of the sick to Ellen, she recognized him (probably through the symbol of the priestly collar) even though she was extremely ill. At that very moment, Ellen became alert, receptive and focused, wanting to participate. She smiled after receiving the sacrament.

We have known for some time that long term memories are embedded deeply in those suffering from Alzheimer's Disease, and are retained more effectively than short term memories. Each confused person is an individual, and knows at deep levels what has been meaningful and what has affirmed his or her uniqueness. The fact that long term memory is relatively unaffected by this disease is one of its few blessings. Rituals are primitive ways to access these long term memories.

Memory accessed in this way has, at its root, a spiritual dimension and a bias towards health. Rituals and feasts provide a sense of the rhythm of the seasons and promote continuity. They sustain the awareness of being rooted in a wider community of identity, and provide an opportunity to express feelings of longing, hope, guilt and gratitude. Through ritual we capture intuitively what is real and recognize spiritual unity with all things.

"Is any one of you sick? He should call the elders of the church to pray over him and anoint him with oil in the name of the Lord. And the prayer offered in faith will make the person well." (James 5:14-16) This biblical passage emphasizes that physical contact is important in healing. Anointing was done in biblical times to designate a person for a particular office or to set aside articles for holy use. In the New Testament, Jesus was anointed with the Holy Spirit. (Acts 10:38) Anointing with oil is one way of physically focusing on the presence of God and becomes a visible outward sign of an inner intention.

Every six months I organize and participate with the priest in a group anointing for the Catholic residents. On the two occasions that this has been done, I have seen similar results. The priest conducting the sacrament of the sick rubs the anointing oil with his fingers in the form of a cross on the forehead and hands of the residents. Even the residents with advanced dementia became focused, reverent and hushed, exhibiting a stilled awareness. Judith is constantly agitated except at hymn sings, other religious services and during these sacramental rituals, when she is calm and attentive. At first I thought it might be a coincidence, but almost two years of observation have confirmed a distinct pattern.

Universal and natural symbolism can stimulate the senses while promoting the mystery that points beyond, to the sacred. Rituals evoke the deep meanings found in significant events and passages. Our experience of life is tied to our bodies and nature. For example, the circle is an important symbol of the cycles of life. It represents the lunar cycle, the menstrual cycle, the cycle of seasons and the other mandalas of the universe. The hymn sings that I conduct on the units are always held in a circle, representing the unending love of God.

Even those who remember little of Christian doctrine have memories of such ritual events as the lighting of the advent wreath (sight), the ashes on Ash Wednesday (touch), the stations of the cross (movement), memories of the palm branches (silence), and the fragrance of the communion wine (smell). These are sensuous bodily experiences which stimulate imagination. In her book, *Reclaiming The Connections*, Kathleen Fischer states that it is at the level of the imagination that we know and experience reality in its wholeness and connectedness.[25] Imagination is sometimes thought to be the realm of children. It is understood as mere fantasy, unreal and unreliable. But I would suggest that imagination is central to a growing spirituality. Pure reason abstracts, while imagination presents things in living colour. When imagination is limited by dementia, any ritual or activity that liberates it becomes a valuable spiritual resource.

Those traditions which were learned earliest are most likely to be retained. Faith symbols, like faith rituals, work in the lives of those suffering from dementia because they reach emotional levels. They do not depend totally on the intellect, and thus it is possible for them to evoke a response. Faith symbols put us in touch with the archetypal stories of the universe. In all the sacraments we express our reliance upon the earth. The universal symbols of fire, light, water, bread, and wine are rich in meaning. Symbols revive our sense of wonder in the ordinary.

Edna reveals some of this power of symbolism. She is now in the end stage of Alzheimer's Disease. As a strong practicing Anglican, her faith has always been an important integrating factor in her life. She was lying in her bed one day, holding the bars on her bed, and rocking back and forth. I wondered if this rocking reminded of her being rocked as an infant, and if this demonstrated her need and desire to be comforted and loved, since she was lying in a near-fetal position. I sat in silence for some time, holding her hand, and then decided to read Psalm 23. Suddenly Edna spoke word-like responses, becoming visibly attentive, focused on my presence. She grabbed my hands firmly with both of hers. No other verbal communication has elicited this type of reaction. Psalm 23 was embedded deeply in Edna's memory, and this memory cue evoked a significant response. It was important to her to hear the familiar words in a world that had become terrifyingly alien. The assurance that God journeys with us through the valley of the shadow of death reminded her that she was not alone. Words such as these can be enormously comforting to one whose total experience has become one of the shadows.

Worship is a call for persons to edify and nurture each other. Paul reminded the first church at Corinth that worship is the primary arena in which to strengthen community (I Cor.1:2 and 14:26). Church and worship are core experiences for many of the confused elderly. A multitude of needs are met in worship. One enters the presence of mystery: the finite seeking the infinite. An sense of security replaces fearfulness. Feelings of belonging, significance and companionship diminish loneliness. The key to ministry with those suffering from dementia lies in expressions of worship which go beyond verbal cues and address spiritual needs.

What can we assume is being transmitted to those with dementia when they view the physical movements which express faith, or when they touch various symbols? The sign of the cross, which traces the height, depth and breadth of God's love, might convey the concept of limitless love which has shared our suffering. Striking the breast might indicate sorrow for sin. The sign of peace could convey God's infinite realm or kingdom of Shalom, of wellbeing and peace. A bowed head or kneeling in prayer indicates reverence for God.

Long services, involved sermons and unfamiliar prayers will not provide experiences of true worship for people with cognitive impairment. But we must not sell them short. Those with mild dementia are receptive to brief reflections using symbols, images or object lessons. People at every level of impairment seem affected by symbols and rituals, music and actions that convey the presence of God. As Israel was reassured in the desert by the pillars of cloud and fire, familiar symbols of God's nearness convey deep reassurance and comfort.

God does not measure our spirituality by our intelligence or by the amount of time spent in prayer. In fact, the Christian scriptures emphasize the necessity of becoming like a child, experiencing God in vulnerability and simplicity. Prayer can occur in a fleeting moment of sincerity, tenderness, or recognition of the Holy.

We should not underestimate the power of the Spirit of God. Caregivers can prompt the faith memory through hymns, prayer, scripture, symbols and nature. Biblical religion cannot be lived apart from matter. Symbols speak deeply to the residents and include such things as snow and snowballs, animals or colourful autumn leaves. Anything that creates a sense of belonging to the community of life and humankind can be a resource for the movement of God's Spirit.

Even play becomes an ingredient in religious life. Holy objects, metaphorical language, stories, physical action, colors, food, and garments of ritual are signals that what is happening is sacred play. David Miller writes in his book, *Gods and Games*, that religious faith itself is play . . . being gripped by a story, a vision, a ritual (game) whose meaning affects one's life pattern and how one sees the world.[26]

No single tool of ministry is effective for every affected person because of individual differences in cognitive ability, the subjective nature of spirituality and the unique interaction between the person with dementia and the caregiver. Only by getting to know each person can the caregiver discover the best avenues of communication.

Joseph Campbell suggests in his book, *Primitive Mythology*, that there are many indications that one of the first symbols humanity used to relate to God was the mother symbol.[27] The mother loves her child because it is hers, life of her life. For the severely impaired, the mother symbol is obviously important in the need for security and love. I have observed often that those with severe Alzheimer's benefit from hugging dolls and teddy bears as transitional objects of love. Indeed we can all benefit from such symbols, especially in times of loneliness, sadness or bereavement. As well, the identity of many older women in long term care facilities has revolved around motherhood. When they lose their sense of themselves as being (or having been) mothers, they are even more confused and anxious. In the article, "To Find A Soul," we find the case study of "Mrs. Jeffries," who seemed fixated on her domestic responsibilities. Following her admission to a care facility she was very distressed. She talked constantly of going home to care for her husband and children. Her husband had been dead for several years and her children were fully grown. Mrs. J. had to be given lorazepam and physically restrained to keep her within the building. Finally, the nurses asked the family to bring in some teddy bears. They brought two beautiful plush bears, one pink and the other blue. Mrs. J. called them "Pinky" and "Blue Boy." They became her children. The nurses reported that she rocked them, bounced them on her lap and talked to them. After the teddy bears arrived, she stopped talking about going home and was able to sit happily in her room, holding the bears in her arms. She could then be removed from the sedative drug. The nurses did not feel that they were treating the resident in a demeaning or condescending manner, as the toys were treated with respect by the staff.[28] In our lives we do receive satisfaction and happiness from the vocations to which God has called us. Experiencing maternal feelings and responsibilities seemed to keep Mrs. Jeffries in tune with the God-call upon her life.

Many cultures recognize in water a symbol for the

naming of the uncontrollable. Water is our first need as living animals. It is our first need in the church as well, and is frequently perceived as a direct gift from God. Water is the source of life and it serves as a profound symbol of the full life. To the Jews of ancient times, who were originally desert nomads, water was a mysterious source of life beyond our supplying. Water was used for ceremonial washings. (Lev.11:32) In modern times, as in biblical contexts, water represents the cleansing of the soul from sin (John 3:5), and is used symbolically in baptism. Our thirst for water is the symbol of our heart's yearning for relationship with God. "As the deer pants for streams of water, so my soul pants for you, O God." (Psalm 42:1) Water represents our connection to the earth, sky and sea.

In a long term care facility, the only contact with water may be a glass of water for drinking and the water used for bathing. There are few opportunities for trips to mountain streams or to the lake or ocean, unless special arrangements are made for field trips. Although such outings may not be economically feasible for those who are severely impaired, tapes are now available which provide an opportunity to listen to pounding ocean surf, splashing waterfalls and gurgling streams. Janine was a resident who expressed a sense of delight at hearing these water sounds when I played such a tape for her. The rippling, liquid sounds of water released in her a deep awareness of the joy in life.

Human beings have always shared meals. Eating together is a symbol of fellowship, common life and love. It is one of the most important activities in the life of a Christian for whom its symbolism is alive. The heart of the worship experience in the Christian tradition is the Eucharist. In Roman Catholicism, to experience the Eucharist is to see, know, feel and even digest God within the framework of the liturgy of eating and drinking. It is an active and social experience. It is an experience of God involving movement and responses. This sacred meal is older than Christianity. Indeed the notion of the sacred meal predated Judaism as well. In primitive societies, the social organism was seen as a single animal with one corporate life blood. The sacred meal became life within the participants and meant partaking of God's very being. When the numinous moments come to those suffering from dementia, as often happens at the Eucharistic meal, we can only imagine what is happening for the worshipper. Helen says that on many occasions she has observed her mother in a state of awe and reverence after Pearl has taken part in the communion meal. These highly specific responses are quite different from her reactions to ordinary life experiences. We can guess from the joy and twinkle in the eye that the worshipper experiences being alive, being in harmony with the rest of creation, and being receptive to the depths of nature and God.

A broad area in need of investigation concerns how to meet the specific religious needs of affected people from other faith backgrounds. Each faith tradition has its own particular symbols, music and rituals that are important to the identity of people from those traditions. Spiritual caregivers of these residents need to know how best to communicate nonverbally to those from a variety of spiritual backgrounds.

We also need more information about meeting the religious and spiritual needs of people who have had no faith background. What songs, symbols, rituals, poetry, images and sensory experiences will serve the spiritual needs of people who have never developed a relationship with the Holy?

In conclusion, my observations and those of the many caregivers I have interviewed affirm that God is experienced through the concrete world by those affected by dementia at levels which cannot be measured, but which nonetheless evoke lucid responses of awe, wonder, reverence and peace in their lives.

TOUCH

From earliest times, the therapeutic power of touch has been recognized in religious thought and in other disciplines. Medicine men, shamans and faith healers have always recognized touch as sacramental, a medium of sacred blessing. The Song of Songs (also called Song of Solomon) is the most sensuous book in the Bible, not only because it celebrates human love and sexuality, but also because it rejoices in the physical experience of the sights, sounds, smells, tastes and textures of creation. Its pages contain descriptions of the delight of human touch, the juice of plump fruits and the aromas of spices and myrrh. Here we have another garden, but one unlike the Garden of Eden where people first experienced shame about their bodies. In this garden, people delight in giving and receiving pleasure. In the early church touch was valued, not just for healing, but also to impart the power of the Holy Spirit.

Touch is a powerful force for wellness. From infancy onwards, affectionate, tactile stimulation is clearly a primary need which must be satisfied in order to develop as a healthy human being. Once past childhood, however, our culture is largely one where touch is uncommon. We enter elevators and immediately place our hands to our sides and look at the floor or indicator lights so as not to touch or even see others. Many people shake hands in greeting only very lightly . Because of our uneasiness with our bodies and bodily needs, we rely heavily on words to convey our thoughts and feelings.

Jesus frequently conveyed his care through touch. He touched lepers, the most untouchable of the afflicted. (Mark 1:41) He laid hands on sick people and touched the eyes of the blind. (John 9:6-7) Jesus hugged children and gave them his blessing. (Mark 10:16) He praised the woman who tenderly anointed him with oil. (John 12:1-8) A woman who had been hemorrhaging for twelve years desired only to touch his clothing, believing that even this minimal contact would be effective for her healing. (Mark 5:25-34) A loving touch may communicate deep feelings that are impossible to express in words. I could cite hundreds of observations of residents for whom a touch brought smiles, tears and joy. Loving touch is a treasured gift to all of us but especially to a person with dementia, who has deep needs for acknowledgement as a unique and treasured person.

Human touch can be a sacrament revealing God's love and healing. It convinces us of our lovableness and beauty. Touch can speak of forgiveness and affection far beyond the scope of language. Touch is multi-dimensional because it can include all aspects of personhood, a deepening consciousness of relationships over time, and feelings of serenity, peace and satisfaction.

Health care professionals are participating more and more frequently in alternative, non-traditional practices within traditional health care settings. The practice of therapeutic touch was developed by Dolores Krieger and Dora Kunz and first described by Krieger in 1973. It is derived from the spiritual practice of the laying on of hands, but differs in that it is not done within a religious context, nor does it require any professed belief by either the practitioner or the recipient. Another difference between therapeutic touch and the laying on of hands is that the former requires no actual physical contact between practitioner and patient. The hands are used to direct energy from the practitioner to the patient with the intent of helping. The conceptual model for therapeutic touch is based on Martha Roger's view of the universe as an open system, with individuals and the environment as energy fields that continually exchange matter and energy.[29]

This way of being present to a person with dementia means taking him or her seriously, listening to their words and sustaining nonverbal communication, even if the process does not make sense to the caregiver. Since the resident with dementia is operating on an emotional plane, rather than an intellectual one, a gentle human touch can be an effective way to reassure the person. A hug will go further than words.

Touch establishes presence and expresses emotion. When Edna grasped my hand after the reading of Psalm 23, her non-verbal communication was at least as important as if she had spoken words to me. Lillian is a resident who finds touch profoundly comforting. Often she takes my hand into hers and gently kisses it. This has happened on other occasions with other residents, and is intensely moving to me. At those moments I feel like the most important person in their world and their gratitude is overwhelming. I have noticed that when I touch a hand or shoulder during a time of prayer, the relationship deepens significantly and there is an exchange of energy. Touch is important for everyone, but was a particular need for Frank. He held both of my hands firmly in his, conveying with his eyes his satisfaction at the human touch.

Edmonton's Shaw Cable aired a documentary program in January 1994, entitled "Alzheimer's: Forgotten Memories," in which I was privileged to take part. My presentation highlighted the importance of spirituality in the care of those with this disease. One of the interviews was with my friend Richard, whose wife Suzanne has been hospitalized for the last seven years. Her condition at that time was already very advanced. When the interviewer asked Richard how he communicated with Suzanne, he simply said, "We hold hands."

AROMA

In a discussion of sensual spirituality, the sense of smell might well be overlooked, particularly since our culture sets such narrow limits around what smells are acceptable.

The Bible mentions incense burning as being symbolic of the ascending prayer of the officiating high priest. The Psalmist prayed, "May my prayer be set before you like incense . . ." (Psalm 141:2a) Revelation 8:3-5, tells of an angel who burns incense on the golden altar from which smoke ascends with the prayers of the saints. Another intriguing scripture says that we are to God the aroma of Christ. (II Cor. 2:15) As we ponder the significance of aroma in scriptures, we discern that God created smell or aroma not only for the pleasure of humankind, but also as a source of pleasure for the

Holy.

The power of smell is profound. It can stir up memories, create moods and change attitudes.[30] Baking sessions are a popular activity on the units of the General Hospital. Enticing aromas from cakes, cookies, pies and other baked goodies, waft through the residents' rooms and the public areas. I have often joined the residents for tea, and have observed them to be much more animated and sociable at these times. Often a resident who has been difficult to get to know in ordinary settings warms up and relaxes into relationship when surrounded by the aroma of home baking.

The fragrance of freshly baked bread or other treats stimulates not only the senses, but also long-ago memories of childhood, with mothers busy in the kitchen. Such memories are pleasurable and life enhancing for the residents. Food aromas also make the facility more homey, which is what having a close relationship with God is like. Experiencing God as loving and unconditionally accepting is a home-like feeling.

I have also chosen to wear a variety of perfumes to stimulate olfactory pleasure, since hospital cleaning agents and the odour of incontinence in a long term care facility can be overpowering at times. Flowers are another source of pleasure; I have often observed residents holding flowers to their nose, soaking in their lovely fragrances. Recently, when she was feeling particularly depressed and hopeless about life, Lillian was able to smile and feel much happier as she breathed deeply the scent of a beautiful bouquet of sweet peas.

One fascinating incident took place following a memorial service I conducted on one of my units. I had brought in some brightly coloured autumn leaves to symbolize the naturalness of the dying process. They were exploding with the intense aroma that many of us recall so vividly from childhood, as we rolled in or hid under great leafy piles. To my surprise, several of the residents reached out their hands at the close of the service for some of the leaves. They not only held them, but wanted to take the leaves back to their rooms. Most intriguing of all, they pulled the leaves to their faces, inhaling deeply to capture the pungent aroma.

Conscious effort is required to offer facility-bound residents the aromas of life. To be taken outside on a spring morning and smell the rain and the loamy earth, to breathe deeply of freshness and new creation, is most restorative. Since the crisp autumn days cannot come to them, they need to be taken out into the coolness, where frost-nipped flowers and burning leaves speak of harvest and completion. Aroma is everywhere, as pervasive as God's presence.

COLOUR

Have you ever begun the day feeling out of sorts? If nothing felt quite right, perhaps you needed a pick-me-up colour for the day. The vibrational energy of colour serves to change one's mood. Colours may even have the power to make people feel better about being alive. Bright colours can inspire, assure and even provide a way of communication with others by the way in which they make the human body visible.

Colour has a long history of meaning which can be traced back through ancient Egypt and the city of Rome, where it was described as one of the resources in the service of health. Pythagoras was reported to have used colour and music to cure disease, while Galen believed that external application of colour could encourage the healing of internal conditions.

The effect of colour on the human mind and body is a subject of increasing interest in in the 1990's. Scientific studies show that red increases the blood pressure, quickens the pulse and increases the rate of breathing. By contrast, blue acts to slow down bodily functions and green has a calming, balancing effect. Notice how fast food outlets use bright oranges and yellows in their decor; orange acts as an appetite stimulant.[31]

Colour, which is reflected light, stimulates mental and emotional responses. Since those affected by dementia are often communicating on an emotional plane, colour becomes another important communication tool. Artists, musicians and philosophers such as da Vinci, Goethe and others, developed theories about the relationships between colour, music and the inner life. Myriad psychiatric studies have led to the development of art therapy which uses colour and form as healing tools in helping patients express hidden emotions. Colours signal and send messages. Folk wisdom attaches specific meanings to certain colours. Red says, "I am strong." Yellow opens communication: "Let's put our hearts together." The favourite of all colours is blue, particularly in technological societies. It is the colour of the intellect and is probably the favoured colour of the left brain. But blue is also known as a colour of remembrance. I often use flowers symbolically at the hymn sings I conduct. Depending on the season, I may have yellow, peach or red blooms. Residents always respond with pleasure.

People with dementia comment on and reach toward strong, bright colours, especially in clothing. These colours seem especially stimulating, increasing alertness and interest. Chaplains (unfortunately conforming to their stereotype!) often tend to wear darker colours. From the delight and interest shown in brightly coloured clothing, it becomes obvious that caregivers can contribute to the happiness of residents by as simple a thing as choosing to wear colourful, visually stimulating clothes.

(At the General Hospital, a master's student conducting research about wandering discovered she had to wear neutral colours in order to avoid drawing attention to herself. The residents' awareness of her presence created a potential for biasing her study.)

Awareness is one of the first steps in an awakened spirituality, and bold colours heighten awareness. Unfortunately, although current research indicates that residents fare better in stimulating surroundings, long term care facilities are frequently painted in pastel shades.

Each summer, during Klondike Days, the city of Edmonton comes down with "goldrush fever." People and businesses indulge in old-time events and costumes. Recently, for the first time in my ministry, I joined in the fun of dressing for the nineties - the 1890's! A chaplain colleague loaned me a full length red dress trimmed with black lace, and a matching red hat with nets and a huge black feather. The responses of the residents, even the severely cognitively impaired, were dramatic. One resident is Irena. In the two years that I have known her I have heard her speak only a few words, always in Ukrainian. Her typical posture is drooped, fixedly gazing into her lap and appearing quite unhappy. When she came to the chapel for the weekly interdenominational service and saw me in my Klondike regalia, she gripped me with both hands and pulled me towards her. It took a great deal of effort to emerge from her solid grasp. But even more surprising than her sudden, enthusiatic grip was her exclamation, in English, of three words: "Dress, hat, funny!" This was followed by a long and hearty laugh. Irena's dramatic reaction prompted me to spend the rest of the day going from unit to unit, visiting many residents to see if it was an individual, isolated response. Resident after resident, whose faces would normally be flat and expressionless, lit up as if they had been awakened from a long sleep. Some tried to touch the lacy sleeve of the flowing dress; many gazed in wonder at the flamboyant hat; all smiled with delight. Perhaps this encounter with someone dressed in 1890's apparel aroused memories from childhood or youth as well.

Recreational therapists who work on the cognitive support unit have reported to me that the residents are quite captivated by brightly coloured balloons and beach balls which they enthusiastically bounce from person to person.

Caregivers could advocate for residents by encouraging builders and maintainers of long term care facilities to paint the interiors in bright and happy shades. God created and maintains this world with a lavish array of colours, wordlessly providing yet another avenue for our enjoyment of the Holy.

PART TWO

SPRITUAL CARE
FOR THE CAREGIVER

CHAPTER 10

EMPOWERING THE CAREGIVER THROUGH SPIRITUALITY

The Hebrew prophet Jeremiah, once said: "If you have raced with men on foot, and they have worn you out, how can you compete with horses? If you stumble in a safe country, how will you manage in the thickets by the Jordan?" (Jeremiah 12:5)

No discussion of spiritual care for those affected by dementia would be complete without discussing the spiritual care of their caregivers. The wellbeing of the affected person is intimately related to the spiritual health of his or her caregiver. Care for the cognitively impaired must be based on relationship rather than task. To sustain the strength to carry on through the multiple years of the dementia condition, and to search for meaning and hope along this arduous journey, one must find a well of energy and nurture.

The most common complaint amongst caregivers is "I am tired." Caring for sufferers of dementia is demanding and socially disruptive, due to the long span of the caregiving task. The caregiver, often a spouse or adult daughter, faces the prospect of isolation, lack of time for self and others, career interruptions, financial drain and unrelieved physical labor, all of which contribute to a sense of burden. For some, it becomes a living hell.

Each person has a story to tell. The Jan.13, 1994 edition of The Edmonton Journal tells of one woman who fought the hopeless battle of keeping her husband at home for eight years. He sometimes got upset if his long dead mother didn't show up for dinner. They stopped watching hockey games because he became afraid that the players would hurt him. When the wife's exhaustion and anxiety became unbearable, she placed him in a long term care facility. This dedicated woman described her emotional pain as "going to hell and back. People have to go through it to understand."[1]

Another caregiver expressed feelings of defeat, stating that she had not run out of power and love, but had lost access to it.

Philosopher John MacMurray asserts that human beings seem to be moved to action by two fundamental motives: love for another and fear for oneself. When applied to caregiving, love for the other moves the caregiver to self transcendence, service and creative management of demands. Fear for oneself, on the other hand, can result in caregivers becoming preoccupied with personal losses and adopting a resistant posture in the face of changes. Fear makes love harder to sustain. Spirituality is a key factor in the empowerment of caregivers and it can help address fear, thus becoming a resource for renewal in the will to care.[2]

Caring for persons affected with dementia can result in stress, guilt and other draining feelings. It requires dealing with losses over and over again. There is anger at the constant demands; hope is difficult to sustain. There is no lack of information about burnout and stress management on the bookshelves. This information provides caregivers with a resource to find ways of coping, but it is not enough. I believe that one needs a more holistic approach, one which sees care-giving as a spiritual endeavor as well as a physical one. Coping mechanisms which support mere survival are not adequate to meet the need for spiritual renewal. My conviction is that our spirituality does more than help us cope, it empowers us.

Pratt, Schmall, Wright and Cleland investigated several coping strategies and reported their findings in a paper entitled, "Burden and Coping Strategies of Caregivers to Alzheimer's Patients." Two hundred and forty subjects were surveyed. Differences in perception of burden were not substantially affected by age, sex, income, education or patient residence. However, burden scores were significantly related to the caregiver's health status and the presence of a support system. The three most common internal coping mechanisms were: confidence in problem solving, ability to reframe the problem and cultivating realistic expectations (technically referred to as "passivity"). Two external coping strategies that were deemed important were spiritual support and the presence of an extended family. Spiritual support, in this context, included the ability to discover the meaning of a problem, the ability to deal with chronic challenges to self-esteem, and skill in clarifying expectations. The authors stated that one's sense of spirituality allows one to neutralize a potential stressor by seeking positive attributes in the situation or by making positive comparisons to others.[3] One respondent commented, "I have never felt resentful of the time caring for my husband, only extremely tired at times. Our love is strong. Our faith is in the Lord." Another said, "This illness is teaching me to gain strength in the Lord. I leave the outcome to God. I am lucky to have my faith." This study found that for those who felt only anger at the situation, meaning was difficult to find.[4] Perhaps this indicates that where meaning is hard to discover, anger becomes the dominant emotion.

Caregiving is about presence and listening. There just isn't always something that we can do. There are many times of helplessness and silence. This is when the caregiver must rely heavily on confidence in his or her own being, a central aspect of a growing spirituality.

There is no one correct way to care for someone who is cognitively impaired. Many factors affect caregiving, including the temperament of the caregiver, the emotional support available to him or her, the caregiver's personal system of beliefs and values, the degree of empathy felt for the recipient of care, and the caregiver's perception of the situation. Though each caregiver is unique, some common traits for those who manage successfully are that they are able to assess difficult situations, are adaptable in the midst of change, have realistic expectations, and are able to determine what can and what cannot be changed or controlled.

Healthy spirituality is characterized by an acceptance of limitations, hope in the face of suffering, and love for its own sake, flowing from the conviction of being unconditionally loved by a God who is always gracious and caring. An unhealthy spirituality is characized by a punitive view of God and life. Caregiving is performed from a sense of duty, with the provider of care unconsciously striving to earn rewards. "Doing" is valued over "being." This can create a situation where stress builds until burnout becomes a real possibility.

The following are some of the factors which can nurture a healthy, empowering spirituality:

1) Maintaining a sense of humour -
   Humour has an energizing power and life giving qualities. It puts our limitations into perspective, and is a deeply spiritual dimension of our being. Accepting our frailties releases the energy we would otherwise use to hide them. This energy can then be applied to the caregiving situation. Humour also tempers anxiety, another energy drainer.

2) Going on pilgrimages rather than vacations -
   Some caregivers don't need vacations as much as they do pilgrimages. Such people are refreshed and energized more by a situation of learning than by empty sightseeing activities. These caregivers need times of renewal, not merely a change of scene.

3) Releasing the energy of both the feminine and the masculine -
   The energy of the masculine is generally defined as taking the initiative to care for the self and dealing efficiently with problems and circumstances. Unless care is creative, the caregiver is likely to lose energy. Creativity breeds energy. Finding nonverbal methods of communicating involves imagination and flexibility. This aspect of our selves is found in what our society generally considers to be the feminine. Both men and women can access both the masculine and feminine aspects of themselves.[5]

4) Entering the pain -
   A growing spirituality allows us to enter the pain, like a dentist enters a cavity to remove decay. Although a very human response, pain avoidance is both futile and enormously draining. The pain of

caring for a beloved person with dementia, when embraced, is like a fuel that provides energy. This energy sensitizes us to the simple and beautiful, makes us more empathic and plumbs the depth of our love and relationships. This is not to glorify pain, but to accept it as part of the human condition, part of the price and privilege of loving, an inevitable aspect of living to be assimilated just as we would take into ourselves the joy and delight that come our way.

5) Tapping into the power of the shadow -
The shadow includes the unwanted qualities in our personalities, which contain a great deal of energy. We access our positive attributes and functions until they are worn out; our shadow side seems chaotic to us, and we fear it. But, for example, anger at the losses caused by dementia can be constructive, motivating us to be advocates for those who live within a world that ignores their needs. Even though the shadow carries the taint of foolishness, it has the power to transform and heal. We can use the shadow with its negative feelings and despised qualities as a reservoir of life, giving energy for caregiving.[6]

6) Nurturing our spirituality type -
A study of spirituality types can be very illuminating. What drives or allures us? What offers us satisfaction and wholeness? This deliberate renewal of our spirits can become a resource for caregiving. Helpful resources might include the Myers-Briggs Type Indicator, the Enneagram, or the book, *Theological Worlds*, by Paul Jones, which details five different theological viewpoints.[7]

7) Drawing upon the energy of symbols -
Jesus described himself in symbols: the door . . . the good shepherd . . . the light. Symbols speak more deeply than words and mobilize and inspire us to greater levels of caring. Symbols which represent the way a caregiver perceives himself or herself, and symbols which represent the way the recipient of care is envisioned, can be life enhancing or draining. If a person is seen as a black lake, devouring energy, the caregiver may be unable to give meaningful time and attention to the other, being preoccupied with self-protection. Constructive, positive symbols energize the caregiver and lead to a renewed perception of the importance of their service.

8) Seeking relationships that support -
The energy drain in caring for others is subtle. Someone has described it as a "slow bleed." Relationships work like photosynthesis. They require energy, but they also give energy. Strength is multiplied when we share in the strength of a supportive community. Supportive people help in three ways: they nourish our souls, they accepts us as we are and they provide safety when we need to be vulnerable. Times of sharing both our successes and the anguish of our struggles often result in more energy for living.

9) Developing a new way of seeing -
To observe someone with dementia is to see something about God. The story of Hagar in Genesis 21 illustrates this point. Hagar was banished into the desert by Sarah's anger and Abraham's indiffer-

ence. She and her child, Ishmael, were lost and without water; Ishmael was close to death. Hagar put the child down, weeping bitter tears. But her broken-hearted cries were heard, and we read, "God opened her eyes so that she saw a well that she had previously not noticed." (Gen. 21:19) With Hagar's new way of seeing, she became aware of God's provision for her and Ishmael. A life that had been full of suffering, in a hopelessly cruel and futile world, was completely changed.

Another example is Christ's experience in the Garden of Gethsemane. After a time of tremendous agony, terror and betrayal, Jesus found the strength and courage to go the way of the cross. Spirituality is more than ethical behavior; it is also a call to see things differently. This reframing of the way we perceive and understand our circumstances can be enlivening.

10) Removing our masks -

When we are being genuine, energy flows in us and from us naturally. To give up any part of our true feelings is to give up a part of ourselves. God works through us as we are unblocked, true to ourselves and vulnerable.₈ Caregiving that is effective and sustainable has to be founded upon a genuine knowledge of self which reveals how we may best care for ourselves. This applies particularly to the areas of limitations and gifts. Clarity of vision helps us to see what is helpful to our wellbeing and what undermines it. People are always in the process of becoming their truest selves. Honesty, with oneself and others, is a basic ingredient for respectful loving relationships.

A healthy spirituality is not frightened by chaos and ambiguity. The person affected by dementia symbolizes chaos to us. When we can walk confidently in their twilight, we discover previously unknown sources of power, joy and wisdom even as we move courageously through the distress. All of the caregivers I have interviewed spoke from amazing places of strength because they overcame the temptation to be crushed by despair. Because they knew their own wounded, vulnerable areas, they had become true channels of God's healing power.

11) Looking through the eyes of hope -
When we face death with hope we release the power of creation into the world. Hope strengthens and sustains. It allows room for a sense of expectation. Hope does not lie in an expectation of improvement, since people with dementia cannot expect to be cured, but it anticipates continued meaning in life and delight in the experiences of living.

Dementia is like the thickets by the Jordan: confusing, entangling and directionless. Within this jungle we find a whole world of suffering. We also realize our own place in it, as we become acutely aware of our limitations and finite capacities to care. But this realization of our humanness, our own need, motivates us in a great journey of discovery, as we seek that which we consider to be our Higher Power.

CHAPTER 11

NETWORKS OF CARE

A t some point, at least fifty percent of the adult population in the United States will care for an aging parent, spouse, sibling or friend. The average time from onset of Alzheimer's Disease until death is 8.1 years. This represents a major span in the lives of an increasing number of people. Caregivers often strive to care for their loved one in the home. This can be a rewarding experience, but acquiring relevant information for unforeseen problems, combating social isolation and maintaining a support network can pose tremendous challenges.

Technologies such as computer networks promise creative new avenues of support and empowerment to caregivers. These networks are designed not for episodic interventions, but for sustained psychosocial support, helping to meet an individual's informational, emotional, or spiritual needs.[1]

The need of caregivers to discuss their feelings and concerns is well known. Family members may be struggling to find meaning in their loved one's suffering. Support groups can be extremely helpful, but the commitment of time and effort required to attend meetings, the logistical problems of obtaining transportation, or the inability to acquire relief caregiving rules out this option for a significant number of people.[2]

A pilot project called Computerlink, dealing with

support of homebound Alzheimer's caregivers, was conducted in Cleveland, Ohio, as a sub-network on the Cleveland public access computer network, Free-Net. Access to Computerlink was limited by password to 47 individuals who were caregivers of persons with Alzheimer's Disease. These individuals had personal computers with modems, enabling them to access Computerlink 7 days a week, 24 hours a day. The caregivers were deemed competent to use the system after ninety minutes of instruction. There were three functions on the system: a communications pathway, an electronic encyclopedia, and a decision support module.[3]

One of the most important features of the system was its 24-hour accessibility. This allowed for psychosocial and spiritual support any time of the day, compared to a traditional group that meets weekly. The mean age of the caregivers was 60.3 years old. Thirty two of the participants were female and fifteen were male. Forty-seven percent were spouses of the care recipients, twenty-nine percent were adult children and thirteen percent were other relatives and friends. The length of the caregiving relationship ranged from four months to ten years.[4]

Emotional support was defined as the expression of sympathy, understanding and a sense of community extended from one caregiver to another. Contrary to popular belief, people did interact on an emotional level, sharing intimate feelings and problems. Spiritual support was defined as the offering of scripture, prayer and inspiration. It was found that psychosocial and spiritual support were demonstrated in varying degrees.

Individuals could use their actual names or remain

anonymous. Since embarrassment and anxiety were often the issues identified when caregivers were asked why they did not participate in traditional support groups, this was highly advantageous. Also, entries could be saved on the network to be retrieved and read again as desired. One member expressed great frustration concerning the financial problems of caregiving and the unavailability of relief support. Within hours, the moderator of the network provided emotional support and empathy, saying, "I'm glad we're able to be here for you. It sounds like you're handling a tough situation pretty well." Another caregiver on the network responded, "We need one another. I'm amazed how we can usually find someone who has a bigger, more difficult situation to cope with than our own. You are all in my prayers." One person said, "simply knowing there are others who understand and take the time to respond is a comfort."5

I.D. Yalom (1985) presents a model of group therapeutic factors. These factors are an instillation of hope, universality, imparting information, altruism, the corrective recapitulation of the primary family group, development of socializing techniques, interpersonal learning, group cohesiveness, catharsis and existential factors. Computerlink participants expressed high satisfaction with this support system because it satisfied all of the Yalom criteria as well as providing 24-hour accessibility.6

There is a national trend to provide health care outside of hospitals, which requires that health caregivers consider nontraditional ways of providing their services. This vision of health care delivery is being shaped quickly in the province of Alberta, and is being directed towards a more community-based model, including such things as Internet access to support groups. It is exciting to anticipate the possibilities of this creative new way to offer psychosocial support to caregivers. This computer network also holds great promise for supporting people in remote areas.

In 1992, a proposal was made in England for the formation of a National Christian Dementia Support Network. This network would express a shared vision that, whether affected by dementia or not, we are all of equal importance in the eyes of God and that we remain fully human beings throughout our lives. It would seek to extend spiritual, pastoral and practical care to caregivers and to people with dementia, giving special emphasis to spiritual and pastoral needs.

In Alberta, as in other Canadian provinces, Alzheimer's Societies have been created which are successfully providing informational services and support groups for caregivers. The proposed English model envisions adding the spiritual component and thus providing a more holistic approach to caregiving. The Alberta Alzheimer's Society provides excellent seminars during their annual Awareness Week and has included spiritual support in these sessions, as well as providing an awareness chapel service as a component of the week. The Society also included the spiritual component in the making of the documentary "Alzheimer's: Forgotten Memories," filmed in January of 1994 by Shaw Cable. In the past, a diagram of the caregiving components (practical, emotional and spiritual) for Alzheimer's patients would have looked something like the following:

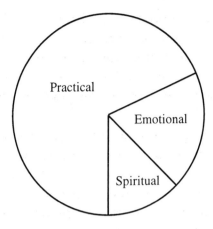

Figure 5

The vision of the English proposal is more holistic, with the components of care modelled as follows:

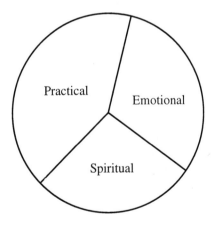

Figure 6

There are three areas which I hope to explore further. The first is investigation into creating a Spiritual Dementia Support Network in Alberta, similar to the one which was proposed in England, but with a broader mandate, encompassing other cultures and faith traditions as well as Christianity. This would extend the efforts of Alzheimer's societies in Canada by raising awareness of dementia in churches and other faith communities.

The second area would be the creation of a computer support network specifically for caregivers of chronically ill people.

The third area is the implementation at the Edmonton General Hospital of a pastoral care course for caregivers of people affected by dementia. Such a course would encourage theological reflection on dementia issues, stimulating both pastoral and practical response.

PART THREE

THE IMPACT
OF SPRITUAL CARE

CHAPTER 12

A NEW IMAGE:
MINISTRY AS RESPONSE TO REALITY

M any times clergy and lay visitors alike have found it difficult to understand the relevance of ministry to the confused elderly. One colleague wanted to know my thesis topic. When I told him it was the spiritual care of those afflicted with dementia, he paused a moment and then responded, "Why?"

If we are unwilling or afraid to scrutinize our biases, prejudices, and assumptions, this type of ministry could well seem irrelevant. To be frank, people affected by dementia are quite unimpressed with theological wisdom. When the ego is subordinated in the process of dementia, tact, politeness and dignity often disappear. Because the ability to deal with abstract and intellectualized faith concepts fades away, the cognitively impaired person may not respond in any tangible way to traditional methods of ministry.

This kind of response can leave the minister feeling unprepared and naked. To be unable to use many of the practical skills of ministry taught in seminary produces great anxiety in some caregivers, and may even impact their professional identity. If one can no longer relate the Christian message with words and abstract concepts, what is left for the cognitively impaired? How can communication about what is Holy and sacred take place?

The loss of identity in the caregiver role that can occur when the intellectual approach becomes impossible is analogous to the experience of those with dementia, who have also lost much of their identity. Both the caregiver and the person with dementia struggle to move from a sense of identity based on skills, abilities and gifts to one based on simply being. In his book, *In The Name Of Jesus*, Henri Nouwen describes this as a "forcing ourselves to reclaim our unadorned self in which we are completely vulnerable, open to give and receive love, irregardless of any accomplishments."[1]

Especially in the later phases of the disease process, those with dementia are often quite unreachable with the current tools of ministry, which appeal primarily to the intellect. This requires a significant change in approach. Instead of providing ministry for passive recipients, the minister supplies the energy and substance of the interaction. The unfamiliarity of pastoral caregivers with this process is a major reason why people with dementia are disenfranchised from their regular congregations. To do effective ministry with the cognitively impaired requires a reframing of the task of ministry. The caregiver, instead of being the expert or the mediator of grace, will have to participate in the world through the recipient's limited vision.

Pastoral care has been described as essentially a listening ministry. But how do we listen to those who have little to say that is rational? Ministry can be full of surprises. A hospital staff member mentioned that at first he thought he was bringing God to the folk he was visiting. Now he believes he is visiting God. Because he has been surprised by the Holy, his visiting is now a privilege rather than simply a religious duty. Matthew 25 says that when we visit one who is sick, we are visiting with Christ. This concept now has more than intellectual interest for him; through the lives of the impaired, it has become woven into the fabric of his own life.

Through my experience in this setting, I have discovered that burnout in caregivers is less likely if they reach out, creatively, to connect in alternate ways. Long term caregivers must see their attempts to communicate as important and worthwhile. One study suggested that caregivers' commitment and attitude were the important factors to the interpretation of cues. Committed caregivers saw the resident as a subject and not as an object.[2]

Spiritual caregiving is the territory of everyone who loves and cares, but the professional spiritual caregiver (minister, rabbi or chaplain) in the institutional setting has an advantage that even family members or friends may not have. While loved ones must deal with grief issues for the person they once knew, the minister in the facility has not known the former self, and is more able to see a full person, albeit one who is confused and complex. While the familial caregiver is dealing with alterations in personality and the grief of decline, they may also be contending with depression, anxiety, physical illness, financial strain and social isolation. These challenges are less likely to affect the professional caregiver whose relationship with the cognitively impaired person is less complex.

Studies have shown that successful problem solving is not significantly related to wellbeing in the caregiver, but there is documented evidence of a correlation between decrease in stress and the use of spirituality as a coping strategy and resource within the relationship.[3]

The article "Alzheimer's Disease in African

American and White Families: A Critical Analysis," speaks to the fact that African families are less likely to use formal support systems, such as institutions, for the care of their loved ones; they rely heavily on informal support such as that which flows from their spirituality. They perceive God in a very personal way, as an integral part of their support system. In a dialogue between caregivers it was noted that when caring became too much to bear, the family members resorted to prayer for strength. The study states that researchers have found that it is an asset when the perception of God is literal and reified.[4]

How do caregivers experience their own spirituality when dealing with dementia? Those who have succeeded in caregiving have discovered a theology that works to bring wholeness to their situation. Faith should to be a resource, not a hindrance. The article, "Emotional Adaptation Over Time in Caregivers for Chronically Ill Elderly People," offers this: thirty-two caregivers of people with Alzheimer's and thirty caregivers of people with metastatic cancer were interviewed three times over two years. Both groups showed a decline in anxiety and negative moods while dementia caregivers also experienced a decline in anger. A self-reported lower strength of religious beliefs explained fifty-four percent of the variance in negative mood, while a higher number of social contacts and strongly self-reported religious faith explained forty-three percent of the variance in positive mood.[5]

Betty was first diagnosed with Alzheimer's Disease in 1988. She still responds to the words, "Jesus," "church" and "God." She is very expressive with her face, her eyes, her smile, and her winks. She leans over to touch and be touched. She draws her visitor's face towards herself. She has a lively sense of humor. Her daughter, Dianne, says that Betty reminds her of the mime clowns who dance. Dianne also related an incident where Betty was on her hands and knees, picking things up from the floor. Betty's husband said she looked like an animal when she did this. In trying to help her father reframe the situation, Dianne asked if there were other options. Was there a better explanation, considering Betty's habits in the past, that would affirm what she was doing rather than judging her? They remembered that Betty had always liked to keep the house clean and appeared to be trying to continue this pattern.

When asked what she had learned from her mother throughout this disease process, Dianne replied that she had learned to value the present, and to trust in the importance of nonverbal communication. She also found courage in the fact that her church maintained a steady relationship with Betty. I asked Dianne where she found God manifested in all of this. She answered that God is always in the today, but that it has helped her to view God through the perspective of time. Prayer gets her through, she said, and also has a sustaining influence on Betty, particularly at bedtime. Dianne has been strengthened by the absolute knowledge of the presence of God, the conviction that there is nowhere one can go that God isn't.

Dianne was emphatic about this. God has a tenacious hold on her mother, for, as she sees it, no one has served God better. Dianne said she needed to let go of her desire to see her mother remembering God, and of her previous judgement that forgetting God is a bad thing. The higher reality is that God loves her mother. Like Helen, with her mother Pearl, this daughter has come to understand that Alzheimer's Disease "just is." We may see it as a bad thing or we can choose to discover in it a blessing. As these caregivers have come to realize, they can take some responsibility for things which will support their mothers' spirituality, but they need not worry about it. Dianne concluded by saying that her mother continues to be her teacher about the nature of God and God's love. She had gained wisdom from what she had formerly thought was foolishness.

Over and over, these caregivers affirm that those with dementia teach us to live fully in the present. In her book, *Winter Grace*, a collection of reflections on growing old creatively, Kathleen Fischer tells Sarah Patton Boyle's story. Boyle was devastated when she realized her favourite cousin, Frank, had Alzheimer's Disease. She could not bear to witness the dimming of his shining mind. Frank had marvellous gifts of laughter, appreciation, imagination and affection. The first lightening of Boyle's darkness came when she saw that his seemingly meaningless struggles were not, in fact, fruitless. They had their own purpose and value, even if they did not fit society's standards of productivity and intelligence.

Boyle said, "I was not successful in holding back the tide of the oblivion that engulfed Frank's mind. But my attitude was new. Now I saw him as the giver and myself as the apprentice."[6] It caused her to cease expending strength on despair. The wiping away of memory allowed him to experience long familiar beauties as though they were fresh from the hand of God. "When we would come on our walks to blooming honeysuckles, or a bed of wild violets, Frank would cry out like a child, 'Oh, look at that,' as though it had never been seen before. Although the past faded quickly, his responses to the present were perceptive and poetic." This experience brought healing for both of them.[7]

This capacity for attentiveness is a rich endowment of the creative God, in whose image we are all made. It is like God's own unwavering attentiveness to everything. "God's eye is on the sparrow . . . not a hair is missed . . ." (Matthew 10:29-31) These forgotten ones can teach us the numinous quality of all creation which we so easily forget. They are a symbol of holy "otherness," a revelation of the hidden face of God.

CHAPTER 13

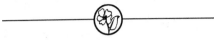

THE PARADOX OF CARING

A strange and powerful paradox occurs when we care for people with dementia. Society prefers to hide them from view. They are an embarrassment to us, and a most disturbing reminder of what we may become in our future years. These people disclose to us our prejudice about what we feel matters in life: knowledge, wealth, prestige, power and energy. They reveal to us the meaninglessness of the very things that we believe give us the most hope for a successful and happy life.

The great paradox in providing their spiritual care is that the one who gives, receives. The one who attempts to bring God to the person with dementia finds God already there, profoundly, in the face and eyes before them. The caregiver, who might put God in an intellectually-perceived theological box, finds God laughing and dancing in the bizarre places where confusion and chaos reign. God is alive in all of creation and no less so among those who are overlooked and ignored by a culture overly dependent on intellect and the verbal articulation of concepts.

The residents I have described comprise a small portion of the cognitively impaired population at the Edmonton General Hospital. Their conditions range from mild to severe dementia. Some have died since I began writing this book. All have touched my life so profoundly that I will never be the same. They have shown me a vision of God. They have stretched me spiritually, exploding my former, limited concepts of where God could reside.

When I first began to visit on a long term care unit, I felt incredible sadness and an overwhelming sense of helplessness and hopelessness. There is a type of culture shock that occurs as the caregiver first experiences this upside down world, where adults can be like infants, where the intellect which is so prized in our society is of minimal importance, where the virtues of childlikeness, simplicity, silence, and living in the present moment are everywhere.

My pastoral helping skills have been more enhanced by this cognitively impaired population than by any other group of people, precisely because the basics of a healthy spirituality are discoverable in their lives. These basics are such things as being childlike, and discovering God in silence, diminishment and suffering as well as in surprise and in the unpredictable. A tremendously important lesson in caregiving emerges from this ministry: becoming more sensitive to others, being inspired and enlightened by feelings, and being open to the natural world are more than just intellectual concepts.

Because of their unpredictable behaviour, caring for people with dementia teaches flexibility and acceptance of failure. Caregivers learn that they cannot spend energy in anticipating what might become of their encounters, but they can revel in the good experiences of the moment, no matter how brief. These moments are celebrated by an emphasis on laughter, music, therapeutic reminiscence, photography and art.

In the experiences that families have shared with

me, and in the example they show daily, I have discovered that the key ingredients to the spiritual care of those affected by dementia are loving commitment to the person, preservation of their dignity, a basic trust in the eternal and unforgetting love of God, and a desire within the caregiver to provide creative experiences that appeal to the soul of the sufferer.

My experiences with these wonderful people have enlivened me with an energy that comes from encountering their faith not in a theoretical way, but in the warp and woof of their living. They are magic mirrors where I have seen my human condition, and have repudiated the commonly held societal values of power and prestige that are unreal and shallow. We have tried to silence the elderly impaired by neglect and indifference, but they can be our most helpful critics and teachers, reflecting to us the inadequacies which we need to address in our values and attitudes. A central change for me has been the overall transformation in how I experience my own spirituality. Those affected by dementia have caused me to develop a deep appreciation of a holistic approach to experiencing God. I have become more nonverbal; I live more in the present; I have become less task oriented and more relational. I have also discovered that we are more than our private memories; we are memories for others and for God. Our very lives are part of a communal memory.

Because people with dementia have their egos stripped from them, their unconscious comes very close to the surface. They, in turn, show us the masks behind which we hide our authentic personhood from the world. We make the elderly with dementia our problem rather than being with them in human solidarity. Visiting people with severe dementia can be an uncomfortable reality for some, forbidding and strange for others. But risking the encounter can lead to the surprise of a new insight. I will never forget the comment of an elderly woman when I asked her about her life experiences. She said, simply, that she had lived an interesting life. After a short pause, she added, "It was full of happiness and unhappiness." It was that simple and true to what life is about.

People with dementia, living in the present and in vulnerability, speak a symbolic language. Their lives are the symbols, revealing what confusion feels like in a life of fear and anxiety, a life without masks that demonstrates the gentleness of childlikeness or the pain of anger and violence. These are places of weakness from a worldly perspective, yet in the Bible we are told that this is where strength is located. (I Cor. 12: 9-10) These so-called weaknesses can be our source of strength and a foundation for relationships. Jesus also lived with the limitations of weakness. (Hebrews 5:2) Accepting weakness in ourselves allows growth in compassion. We can make positive use of religion to bring about an operational theology that serves the specific needs of the cognitively impaired without attempting to deny the impairment or change the person.

The cognitively impaired elderly help us confront the greatest fear of all, that of our own aging and death. Coming to terms with death is difficult, because we may feel we have squandered life or not rectified our wrong doings. People with dementia help us see that God does not condemn us for our incompleteness. If developing integrity and overcoming despair is the task of the elderly, then it is also the task of the caregiver to accept the life situation of the loved one as the only one presently available for them. Death is always a leap into the unknown. The Christian promise of resurrection locates continuity in the steadfastness of God, not in human indestructibility. It takes trust to believe that God's surprises will be in our favour when we die. Ministering with those affected by dementia teaches us about realistic hope; life can be lived fully at any age and in any state. In some inexplicable manner, the mystery of dementia has changed my life and made me healthier. In the words of St. Paul, ". . . God's foolishness is wiser than human wisdom and God's weakness is stronger than human strength." (I Cor. 1:25)

We feel naked before the mystery of life. We prefer to imagine the future as uninterrupted, free of unpleasant surprises, and always under our control. This is an illusion; life is not like that. Living with dementia is living with unpredictability, instability and discontinuity on a grand scale. The usual props are gone. The awareness of vulnerability makes trusting a matter of survival. These are invaluable lessons for the caregiver.

Maturity does not come from repeatedly choosing familiar paths, but from risking those that explode our concepts and preconceptions. In these very difficult and often startling experiences we are forced to receive gifts that we may have shunned as dangerous and disruptive in the past.

I began this book by saying that people affected by dementia are symbolically like the winter season, showing us things we cannot see in the lush undergrowth of the summer of our lives. Macrina Wiederkehr in her book, *A Tree Full Of Angels*, draws this image: "I love the way winter stands there saying, I dare you not to notice my beauty. What can I say to a winter tree when I am able to see the shape of its soul, because it has finally let go of its protective leaves? What can you say to an empty tree? Standing before an empty tree is like seeing it for the first time. Oh, the things that you can see when you are empty."[1]

Winter is still my least favorite season. But although I resist it strenuously because of my reluctance to learn its tough lessons, I need its harshness to teach me endurance and hope. Dementia is a long harsh winter. It has been a difficult journey for me to accept the dementia season in my grandmother's life. Grammie McCloskey never became great or famous in any worldly sense. She was a lovely, diminutive woman who worked hard all the days of her life. Dementia seemed to empty her of all but the core of her soul, which remained to her last days as a core of pure kindness and gentleness.

But true greatness appears in many unexpected guises. M. Scott Peck, in his book *People Of The Lie*, says that stress is the test of goodness. The truly good are those who in times of stress do not desert their integrity, their maturity, their sensitivity . . . Nobility might be defined as the capacity not to regress to degradation, not to become blunted in the face of pain, to tolerate the agonizing and remain intact . . . One measure and perhaps the best measure of a person's greatness is the capacity for suffering.[2]

When I read Peck's definition of greatness, I feel a huge "YES!" arising in my spirit. My research and reflection have helped me to see the shape of Grammie McCloskey's soul even more clearly than I did as a child. Grammie's noble vocation as a young and middle-aged woman was to love and raise her family. Her vocation in later years seems to have been one of suffering. Uniting her sufferings with those of Christ, I have begun to see what made her truly great. She was not blunted in the face of pain. My words to Grammie at this moment are, "Thank you for filling my spirit with your inspiration. I love you Grammie. I love you for your bravery in living through the experience of becoming empty."

My friend, Helen, shares this poem written for her mother by a friend, Linda Long.

HAZEL

You were trying to pry the door open
when we arrived.
As you turned in response
to my touch,
Your face was upset and confused
for a moment
until you saw the faces of my
two small boys
whose job we had told them
was to hug.
Arms outstretched you reached
for their smiles,
kisses, hugs, happiness, warmth
cleansed your face.
"A little music?" "Oh, my, yes,
that would be nice."
Arms linked we strolled past many
other faces.
Out the door that frustrated you,
into song.
You sat, he played, your face,
entered the music.
Body moving, ear turned to hear,
feet moving.

"Hazel, would you like to dance?"
"Oh, would I ! "
Sure footed, strong rhythm, I let you lead me.
And for one second I looked
into your soul.
You did not know at the moment
who I was;
You did not know where you were,
who you were.
But at that beautiful moment
you were beauty,
you were love,
you were music,
you were life,
you were dancing!

by Linda Long
(15 October 1990)

To rejoice in ministry amongst those with dementia requires a special realization that it is relevant. In a world where perhaps the majority of people do not recognize or remember God in daily life, such a ministry has vital implications. The caregiver must do better what all of us should do well: wait actively, remember gratefully, hope realistically, and trust courageously.

When we can see and recognize God behind all the forgetful faces, respond to God in people who are unconscious of the Holy, and point to God in all people, we will have absorbed some of the lesson that cognitively impaired people offer us.

APPENDICES
ENDNOTES
BIBLIOGRAPHY

APPENDIX A

DEFINITION OF TERMS

In the course of this book, a number of technical and theological terms have been used fairly frequently. The definitions of those terms, unless otherwise stated in the text, are as follows:

Dementia: A word to describe the mental condition of a person affected by any neurological disease that results in confusion, loss of memory and loss of intellectual abilities.

Spiritual: "The 'life force' springing from within us all that pervades our entire beings, and includes the emotional, the ethical, the social, the intellect and the physical dimensions."[1] "It is that which gives meaning, purpose and direction in life. It may be understood in a religious, philosophic and humanistic sense."[2]

Religious: "That which pertains to an organization or system of thought which believes in the existence of the divine, that must be worshipped and obeyed."[3]

Spiritual Care: "Care which searches to discover and nurture the inner person and the framework of meaning and values through which it is expressed."[4]

Long Term Care: Represents the stage in the older person's life when one can no longer live independently. It is where familiar surroundings and broad mobility are replaced by a highly circumscribed environment. Frailty is everywhere in the institution, thereby increasing the threat and pressure of death. For the majority of residents, cognitive abilities are (or will become) minimal. Thus the spiritual needs of the elderly in long term care facilities have a special urgency and poignancy, that in turn, poses many challenges for those ministering to them or simply working within these settings.

Need: "A condition, deficiency or distress that requires some extraneous aid or action."[5]

Faith Community: "A group of people who share a common understanding and/or belief about the purpose or meaning of life, whether or not such an understanding includes a supernatural component."[6]

Support Community: "The individuals and groups upon which a person can rely to give social, economic, physical, emotional, intellectual, and/or spiritual support during times of stress. This support may or may not include family members."[7]

APPENDIX B

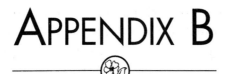

THE ALZHEIMER'S PRAYER

Dear God,

    We pray:

For those who have died of Alzheimer's Disease,
        peace,
For those who are victims of Alzheimer's Disease,
        dignity and comfort,
For the Alzheimer's caregivers,
        compassion and patience,
For the Alzheimer's families,
        strength and courage,
For those who seek the cause,
    cure, prevention, and
    treatment of Alzheimer's,
        your guidance and direction.

For the hope you have given us,
        our thanks.
Amen.

                        Anonymous

ENDNOTES

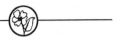

PART ONE - SPIRITUAL CARE FOR THE AFFLICTED

CHAPTER 2
THE NATURE OF DEMENTIA

[1] Morley Jahrig, "A Caregiver Shares His Thoughts, Edmonton," *People and Progress Magazine,* Capital Care Group, May/June 1994.

[2] Nancy Millar, *I Think I Should Know These Trees,* Calgary: Deadwood Publishing, 1993.

[3] D. Dungee-Anderson, et al., "Alzheimer's Disease in African- American and White Families: A Clinical Analysis," *The Smith College Studies in Social Work,* Vol. 62(2), March 1992, pp. 155-168.

[4] Edward Hayes, *Prayers For A Planetary Pilgrim,* Leavenworth, Kansas: Forest of Peace Books Inc., 1989, p. 15.

[5] "Seniors Alive: The Challenge to the Religious Community and the Helping Professions." Proceedings of the Spiritual Well-Being of the Elderly Conference, Edmonton, Alberta. June, 1981.

[6] Marty Richards, "The Challenge of Maintaining Spiritual Connectedness with Persons Institutionalized with Dementia," *The Journal of Religious Gerontology,* Haworth Inc., Vol.7(3), 1991, p. 27.

CHAPTER 3
AN IMAGE: THE CHURCH AS
SUFFERING WITH SENILE DEMENTIA

[1] *The Edmonton Journal*, Nov. 13, 1993: David Briggs, "The Elderly Cope Better with Belief in God."

CHAPTER 4
SPIRITUAL CARE AND MODELS OF AGING

[1] Matthew Fox, *Original Blessing*, Santa Fe, New Mexico: Bear & Company, 1983, p. 35.

[2] Ibid, p. 35.

[3] Moira Reinhardt, "My Spirit Greets Your Spirit," *Nursing Home*, July/August 1991, p. 32.

[4] Harold Kushner, *Who Needs God?* New York: Pocket Books, 1989, p. 170.

[5] James N. Lapsley, "Practical Theology and Pastoral Care: An Essay in Pastoral Theology," *Practical Theology*, ed. Donald S. Browning, San Francisco: Harper & Row, 1983, p. 184.

[6] Ronna Jevne, *It All Begins With Hope*, San Diego, California: LuraMedia, 1991.

[7] Thomas St. James O'Connor, "Ministry Without A Future," *The Journal of Pastoral Care*, Vol. 1, 46, No. 1, Spring 1992, pp. 6-10.

[8] Charles V. Gerkin, "Pastoral Care and Models of Aging," *The Journal of Religion and Aging*, Vol. 6, No. 3/4, 1989, pp. 85-88, cited by Paul W. Pruyser, "Aging: Downward, Upward, or Forward," *Toward a Theology of Aging*, ed. Seward Hiltner, New York: Human Science Press, 1975, pp. 102-118.

[9] Ibid, 85-88.

[10] Ibid, 92-94.

[11] Victor Frankl, *Man's Search for Meaning*, New York: Pocket Books, 1959, p. 161.

[12] Kathleen Fischer, *Winter Grace*, New York: Paulist Press, 1985, p. 111.

[13] Gerkin, pp. 94-95.

[14] Ibid, pp. 94-95.

[15] O'Connor, p. 5.

[16] Gerkin, pp. 95-99.

[17] S.L. Ekman, et al., "Care of Demented Patients with Severe Communication Problems," *Scand J Caring Sci*, Vol. 5, No. 3, 1991, p. 169.

[18] Ibid, p. 163.

[19] Coplan Consultants, *Spiritual Wellbeing in Long Term Care, A Report on the Chaplaincy Demonstration Program at Capital Care (Dickensfield), North Vancouver*, June 1993, pp. 124-127.

[20] Patricia Brown Couglan, *Facing Alzheimer's*, New York: Ballantine Books, 1993, p. 1.

[21] S.L. Scally, et al., "Dignity: The Cornerstone of Care," *Caring Magazine*, Dec. 1991, pp. 45-49.

CHAPTER 5
THEOLOGICAL REFLECTION

[1] Eugene C. Bianchi, *Aging As A Spiritual Journey*, New York: Crossroad, 1987, p. 175.

[2] Ibid, p. 181.

[3] Pierre Teilhard de Chardin, *The Divine Milieu*, New York: Harper & Row, 1960, p. 67.

[4] Paul Wilson, "Dementia: A Christian Response," *The Road To Greater Understanding*, CCOA Conference, April 24-25, 1992, p. 2.

[5] de Chardin, p. 76.

[6] *The Vancouver Sun*, Nov. 1992: Rick Pedersen, "Gardens Found to Soothe Alzheimer's Patients."

[7] *The Edmonton Journal*, Jan. 13, 1994: "New $2.5 M. Residence to be Built for Victims of Alzheimer's Disease."

[8] Thomas Moore, *Care of the Soul*, New York: Harper Perennial, 1994, pp. 126-127.

[9] *The Edmonton Journal*, June 16, 1993: Gordon Kent, "Student Takes New Look at Old Problem."

[10] Ibid.

[11] *The Edmonton Journal*, Nov. 3, 1992: "Dusk to Dawn."

[12] Kushner, p. 182.

[13] W. Harold Grant, et al., *From Image to Likeness*, New York: Paulist Press, 1983, p. 30.

[14] O'Connor, p. 10.

[15] Paul Pruyser, *The Minister as Diagnostician*, Philadelphia, PA: Westminister, 1976, pp. 64-66.

[16] O'Connor, p. 10.

[17] Fischer, p. 127.

CHAPTER 6
SPIRITUAL ASSESSMENT

[1] G. Stoddard, et al., *Developing an Integrated Approach to Spiritual Assessment: One Department's Experience*, p. 65.

[2] Ibid, p. 71.

[3] Ibid, p. 71.

CHAPTER 7
ISSUES OF GRIEF AND LOSS

[1] E. LaBarge, et al., "Counseling Clients with Mild Senile Dementia of the Alzheimer's Type," *The Journal of Neuro Rehabilitation*, Vol. 2, No. 4, 1988, p. 167.

[2] Ibid, p. 168.

[3] Ibid, pp. 169-170.

[4] Scally, et al., pp. 45-49.

[5] Martha O. Adams, *Alzheimer's Disease*, St. Meinrad, Indiana: Abbey Press, 1986, p. 90.

CHAPTER 8
THE ROLE OF REMINISCENCE

[1] Robert L. Randall, "Reminiscing in the Elderly: Pastoral Care of Self Narrative," *The Journal of Pastoral Care*, Vol. XV, No. 3, Sept. 1986, p. 207.

[2] Ibid, p. 207.

[3] Robert N. Butler, "The Life Review: An Interpretation of Reminiscence in The Aged," *Psychiatry*, Vol. 26, 1963, pp. 63-76.

[4] Randall, p. 207.

[5] Mary Lashley, "Reminiscence: A Biblical Basis for Telling Our Stories," *The Journal of Christian Nursing*, Summer 1992, pp. 5-8.

[6] Sandra Martz, ed., *When I Am An Old Woman I Shall Wear Purple*, Watsonville, California: Papier Mache Press, 1991, p. 169.

CHAPTER 9
ALTERNATE METHODS OF SPIRITUAL CARE

[1] Fox, p. 36.

[2] Lois J. McCloskey, "The Silent Heart Sings," *Generations (Counseling and Therapy)*, Winter 1990, p. 65.

[3] J.M. Cohen, "Rhythm and Tempo in Mania," *Music Therapy*, Vol 6A(1), 1986, pp. 41-56.

[4] Helen Bonny Lindquist, "Music and Healing," *Music Therapy*, Vol. 6A(1), 1986, pp. 3-12.

[5] Joan Butterfield Whitcomb, "Thanks for the Memory," *The American Journal of Alzheimer's Care and Related Disorders Research*, July/August 1989, p. 32.

[6] J.W. Ellor, et al., "Ministry with the Confused Elderly," *The Journal of Religion and Aging*, Haworth Press, Vol. (2), 1987, pp. 27-30.

[7] Whitcomb, p. 32.

[8] Nahama Glynn, "The Music Therapy Assessment Tool," *The Journal of Gerontological Nursing*, Vol. 18(1), 1992, pp. 3-9.

[9] A. Clair, et al., "Preliminary Study of Music Therapy in Programming for Severely Regressed Persons with Alzheimer's Type Dementia," *The Journal of Applied Gerontology*, A(9), 1990, pp. 299-311.

[10] K. Millard, et al., "The Influence of Group Singing Therapy on the Behavior of Alzheimer's Patients," *The Journal of Music Therapy*, (26), 1989, pp. 58-70.

[11] C. Prubett, et al., "The Use of Music to Aid Memory of Alzheimer's Patients," *The Journal of Music Therapy*, (28), 1991, pp. 101-110.

[12] Lucanne Magill Bailey, "The Effects of Live Music Versus Tape-Recorded Music on Hospitalized Cancer Patients," *The Journal of Music Therapy*, Vol. 3, No. 1, 1993, pp. 17-28.

[13] McCloskey, p. 63.

[14] Lindquist, p. 8.

[15] McCloskey, p. 63.

[16] Lucanne Magill-Lavreault, "Music Therapy in Pain and Symptom Management in Music Therapy," *The Journal of Palliative Care*, 9:4, 1993, pp. 37-55.

[17] Rachel Mavely, "Consider Karaoke," *The Canadian Nurse*, Jan. 1994, p. 23.

[18] Thomas Moore, *Soulmates*, New York: Harper-Collins Publications, 1994, p. 171.

[19] Fox, p. 227.

[20] J. Bailey RN, et al., "To Find A Soul," *Nursing*, July 1992, pp. 63-64.

[21] Ibid, pp. 63-64.

[22] Hayes, pp. 282-285.

[23] Adams, p. 81.

[24] Ibid, pp. 83-84.

[25] Kathleen Fischer, *Reclaiming the Connections*, Kansas City, Mo.: Sheed & Ward, 1990, p. 13.

[26] David L. Miller, *God and Games: Toward A Theology of Play*, New York: Harper & Row, 1973, p. 168.

[27] Joseph Campbell, *Primitive Mythology*, London: Penquin Books, 1969.

[28] Bailey, et al., pp. 63-64.

[29] Nelda Samarel, "The Experience of Receiving Therapeutic Touch," *The Journal of Applied Nursing*, (17), 1992, pp. 651-657.

[30] Hayes, p. 239.

[31] Dorothee L. Mella, *The Language of Color*, New York: Warner Books, 1988, 1-17.

PART TWO - SPIRITUAL CARE FOR THE CAREGIVER

CHAPTER 10
EMPOWERING THE
CAREGIVER THROUGH SPIRITUALITY

[1] *The Edmonton Journal*, Jan. 13, 1994: "New $2.5 M. Residence to be Built for Victims of Alzheimer's Disease. "

[2] Don Meisener, "A Spirituality That Empowers Caregiving, " Presentation made at the Saskatchewan Association of Health Organizations Convention, Regina, Saskatchewan, Oct. 29, 1993.

[3] C.C. Pratt, et al., "Burden and Coping Strategies of Caregiving of Alzheimer's Patients and Family Relations," 1985, 34, pp. 27-33.

[4] Ibid, p. 31.

[5] John A. Sanford, *Ministry Burnout*, New York: Paulist Press, 1982, p. 30.

[6] Anthony Storr, ed., *The Essential Jung*, Princeton, N.J.: Princeton University Press, 1983, pp. 91-93.

[7] W. Paul Jones, *Theological Worlds*, Nashville: Abingdon Press, 1989.

[8] Sanford, pp. 72-77.

CHAPTER 11
NETWORKS OF CARE

[1] P.F. Brennan, et al., "Computerlink: Electronic Support for the Home Caregiver," *Adv Nurs Sci*, Aspen Publishers Inc., 13(4), 1991, pp. 14-27.

[2] Ibid.

[3] P.F. Brennan, et al., "A Nursing Medium: Computer Networks for Group Intervention," *The Journal of Psychosocial Nursing,* Vol. 30, No. 7, 1992, pp. 15-20.

[4] R.L. Gallienne, et al., "Alzheimer's Caregivers: Psychosocial Support Via Computer Networks," *The Journal of Gerontological Nursing,* Dec. 1993, pp. 5-22.

[5] Ibid.

[6] P.F. Brennan, et al., *The Journal of Psychosocial Nursing,* Vol. 30, No. 7, 1992, pp. 18-19.

PART THREE - THE IMPACT OF SPIRITUAL CARE

CHAPTER 12
A NEW IMAGE:
MINISTRY AS RESPONSE TO REALITY

[1] Henri Nouwen, *In The Name of Jesus: Reflections on Christian Leadership,* New York: Crossroads, 1989.

[2] Scally, et al., pp. 45-49.

[3] P.V. Rabins, et al., "Emotional Adaptation Over Time in Caregivers for Chronically Ill Elderly People," *Age and Ageing,* Vol 19, 1990, pp. 185-190.

[4] Dungee-Anderson, et al., pp. 155-168.

[5] Rabins, et al., pp. 185-190.

[6] Fischer, *Winter Grace,* pp. 110-111.

[7] Ibid, pp.110-111.

CHAPTER 13
THE PARADOX OF CARING

[1] Macrina Wiederkehr OSB, *A Tree Full of Angels*, San Francisco: Harper Collins Publishers, 1990, p. 93.

[2] M. Scott Peck, *People of the Lie*, New York: Simon & Schuster, 1983, p. 222.

APPENDIX A
DEFINITION OF TERMS

[1] Madalon O'Rawe Amenta and Nancy Bohnet, *Nursing Care of the Terminally Ill*, Boston: Little, Brown, 1986, p. 116, as quoted in Amenta 1988, p.48, and Madalon O'Rawe Amenta, "Nurses as Primary Spiritual Care Workers," *The Hospice Journal*, 4 , No. 3, 1988, pp. 47-55.

[2] Patricia Anne Randolph Flynn, *Holistic Health: The Art and Science of Care*, Bowie, Maryland: Robert J. Brady, 1980, p. 12.

[3] Amenta, p, 118.

[4] Ibid, p. 117.

[5] Ibid, p. 8.

[6] Patricia Seale, "Pastoral Care as Spiritual Care," Edmonton: St. Stephen's College, 1990, p. 6.

[7] Ibid, p. 7.

BIBLIOGRAPHY

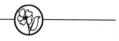

Adams, Martha O. *Alzheimer's Disease*. St. Meinrad, Indiana: Abbey Press, 1986.

Amenta, Madalon O'Rawe. "Nurses as Primary Spiritual Care Workers." *The Hospice Journal*, 4, No. 3, 1988.

Amenta, Madalon O'Rawe: and Bohnet, Nancy. *Nursing Care of the Terminally Ill*. Boston: Little Brown, 1986.

Bailey, J., RN; Gilbert, E., RN; and Herweyer, S., RN. "To Find A Soul." *Nursing*, July 1992.

Bianchi, Eugene C. *Aging as a Spiritual Journey*. New York: Crossroad, 1987.

Brennan, P.F.; Moore, S.M.; and Smyth, K.A. "Computerlink: Electronic Support for the Home Caregiver." *Adv Nurs Sci*, Aspen Publishers Inc., 13(4), 1991.

Brennan, P.F.; Ripich, S.; and Moore, S.M. "A Nursing Medium: Computer Networks for Group Intervention." *The Journal of Psychosocial Nursing*, Vol 30, No. 7, 1992.

Butler, Robert N. "The Life Review: An Interpretation of Reminiscence." *The Aged In Psychiatry*, Vol. 26, 1963.

Butterfield Whitcomb, Joan. "Thanks for the Memory." *The American Journal of Alzheimer's Care and Related Disorders Research*. July/August 1989.

Campbell, Joseph. *Primitive Mythology*. London: Penguin Books, 1969.

Clair, A.; and Bernstein, B.A. "Preliminary Study of Music Therapy in Programming for Severely Regressed Persons with Alzheimer's Type Dementia." *The Journal of Applied Gerontology*, A(9), 1990.

Cohen, J.M. "Rhythm and Tempo in Mania." *Music Therapy*, Vol. 6A(1), 1986.

Coplan Consultants. *Spiritual Wellbeing in Long Term Care; A Report on the Chaplaincy Demonstration Program at Capital Care (Dickensfield), North Vancouver.* June 1993.

Couglan, Patricia Brown. *Facing Alzheimer's.* New York: Ballantine Books, 1993.

de Chardin, Pierre Teilhard. *The Divine Milieu.* New York: Harper & Row, 1960.

Denizen, N.K. *On Understanding Emotion.* San Francisco: Jossey-Bass, 1984.

Dungee-Anderson, D. and Beckett, J. "Alzheimer's Disease in African-American and White Families: A Clinical Analysis." *Smith College Studies in Social Work,* March, Vol. 62(2), 1992.

Eisner E.W. "On the Difference Between Scientific and Artistic Approaches to Qualitative Research." *Educational Researcher*, 10(4), 1981.

Ekman, S.L.; Norberg, A.; Viitanen, M.; and Winblad, B. "Care of Demented Patients with Severe Communication Problems." *Scand J Caring Sci*, Vol. 5, No. 3, 1991.

Ellor, J.W.; Stettner, J.; and Spath, H. "Ministry with the Confused Elderly." *The Journal of Religion and Aging*, Haworth Press, Vol. 4(2), 1987.

Fischer, Kathleen. *Reclaiming the Connections.* Kansas City, MO.: Sheed & Ward, 1990.

Fischer, Kathleen. *Winter Grace.* New York: Paulist Press, 1985.

Flynn, Patricia Anne Randolph. *Holistic Health: The Art and Science of Care.* Bowie, Maryland: Robert J. Brady, 1980.

Fox, Matthew. *Original Blessing.* Santa Fe, New Mexico: Bear & Company, 1983.

Frankl, Victor. *Man's Search for Meaning.* New York: Pocket Books, 1959.

Gallienne, R.L.; Moore, S.M.; and Brennan, P.F. "Alzheimer's Caregivers: Psychosocial Support Via Computer Networks." *The Journal of Gerontological Nursing,* Dec. 1993.

Gerkin, Charles V. "Pastoral Care and Models of Aging." *The Journal of Religion and Aging,* Vol. 6, No. 3/4, 1989.

Glynn, Nahama. "The Music Therapy Assessment Tool." *The Journal of Gerontological Nursing,* Vol. 18(1), 1992.

Grant, W. Harold; Thompson, Magdala; and Clarke, Thomas E. *From Image to Likeness.* New York: Paulist Press, 1983.

Hayes, Edward. *Prayers For A Planetary Pilgrim.* Leavenworth, Kansas: Forest of Peace Books Inc., 1989.

Jahrig, Morley. "A Caregiver Shares His Thoughts, Edmonton." *People and Progress Magazine,* Capital Care Group, May/June 1994.

Jevne, Ronna. *It All Begins With Hope.* San Diego, California: LuraMedia, 1991.

Jones, W. Paul. *Theological Worlds*. Nashville: Abingdon Press, 1989.

Kushner, Harold. *Who Needs God?* New York: Pocket Books, 1989.

LaBarge, E.; Rosenman, L.S.; Leavitt, K.; and Christiani, T. "Counseling Clients with Mild Senile Dementia of the Alzheimer's Type." *The Journal of Neuro Rehabilitation*, Vol. 2, No. 4, 1988.

Lapsley, James N. "Practical Theology and Pastoral Care: An Essay in Pastoral Theology." *Practical Theology*, ed. Donald S. Browning. San Francisco: Harper & Row, 1983.

Lashley, Mary. "Reminiscence: A Biblical Basis for Telling Our Stories." *The Journal of Christian Nursing*, Summer 1992.

Lincoln, Y.S. and Guba, E.G. *Naturalistic Inquiry*. Beverley Hills: Sage Publications, 1985.

Lindquist, Helen Bonny. "Music and Healing." *Music Therapy*, Vol. 6A(1), 1986.

Magill Bailey, Lucanne. "The Effects of Live Music Versus Tape-Recorded Music on Hospitalized Cancer Patients." *The Journal of Music Therapy*, Vol. 3, No. 1, 1993.

Magill-Lavreault, Lucanne. "Music Therapy in Pain and Symptom Management in Music Therapy." *The Journal of Palliative Care*, 9:4, 1993.

Martz, Sandra, ed. *When I Am An Old Woman I Shall Wear Purple*. Watsonville, California: Papier Mache Press, 1991.

Mavely, Rachel. "Consider Karaoke." *The Canadian Nurse,* Jan. 1994.

McCloskey, Lois J. "The Silent Heart Sings." *Generations (Counseling and Therapy),* Winter 1990.

Meisener, Donald. "A Spirituality That Empowers Caregiving." Presentation made at the Saskatchewan Association of Health Organizations Convention, Regina, Saskatchewan, Oct. 29, 1993.

Mella, Dorothee L. *The Language of Color.* New York: Warner Books, 1988.

Merriam, S.B. *Case Study Research in Education; A Qualitative Approach.* San Francisco: Jossey-Bass, 1988 .

Millar, Nancy. *I Think I Should Know These Trees.* Calgary: Deadwood Publishing, 1993.

Millard, K. and Smith, J. "The Influence of Group Singing Therapy on the Behavior of Alzheimer's Patients" *The Journal of Music Therapy,* (26), 1989.

Miller, David L. *God and Games: Toward A Theology of Play.* New York: Harper & Row, 1973.

Moore, Thomas. *Care of the Soul.* New York: Harper Perennial, 1994.

Moore, Thomas. *Soulmates.* NewYork: Harper-Collins Publications, 1994.

Nouwen, Henri. *In The Name of Jesus: Reflections on Christian Leadership.* New York: Crossroads, 1989.

O'Connor, Thomas St. James. "Ministry Without A Future." *The Journal of Pastoral Care,* Vol. 1, 46, No. 1, Spring 1992.

Patton, M.Q. *Qualitative Evaluation and Research Methods.* London: Sage Publications, 1990.

Peck, M. Scott. *People of the Lie.* New York: Simon & Schuster, 1983.

Pratt, C.C.; Schmall, V.L.; Wright, S.; and Cleland, M. "Burden and Coping Strategies of Caregiving of Alzheimer's Patients and Family Relations." 34, 1985.

Prubett, C.; and Moore, R. "The Use of Music to Aid Memory of Alzheimer's Patients." *The Journal of Music Therapy,* 28, 1991.

Pruyser, Paul W. "Aging: Downward, Upward, or Forward." *Toward a Theology of Aging,* ed. Seward Hiltner. New York: Human Science Press, 1975.

Pruyser, Paul W. *The Minister as Diagnostician.* Philadelphia, PA: Westminister, 1976.

Rabins, P.V.; Fitting, M.D.; Eastham, J.; and Zabora, J. "Emotional Adaptation Over Time in Caregivers for Chronically Ill Elderly People." *Age and Ageing,* Vol. 19, 1990.

Randall, Robert L. "Reminiscing in the Elderly: Pastoral Care of Self Narrative." *The Journal of Pastoral Care,* Vol. XV, No. 3, Sept. 1986.

Reinhardt, Moira. "My Spirit Greets Your Spirit." *Nursing Home,* July/August 1991.

Richards, Marty. "The Challenge of Maintaining Spiritual Connectedness with Persons Institutionalized with Dementia." *The Journal of Religious Gerontology,* Haworth Inc., Vol. 7(3), 1991.

Samarel, Nelda. "The Experience of Receiving Therapeutic Touch." *The Journal of Applied Nursing,* 17, 1992.

Sanford, John A. *Ministry Burnout.* New York: Paulist Press, 1982.

Scally, S.L.; Woodridge, P.; and Daum, G. "Dignity: The Cornerstone of Care." *Caring Magazine,* Dec. 1991.

Seale, Patricia. *Pastoral Care as Spiritual Care.* St. Stephen's College: Edmonton, 1990.

Stoddard, G. and Burns-Haney, J. *Developing an Integrated Approach to Spiritual Assessment: One Department's Experience.*

Storr, Anthony, ed. *The Essential Jung.* Princeton, N.J.: Princeton University Press, 1983.

The Edmonton Journal, Nov. 3, 1992: "Dusk to Dawn."

The Edmonton Journal, June 16, 1993: Kent, Gordon, "Student Takes New Look at Old Problem."

The Edmonton Journal, Nov.13, 1993: Briggs, David, "Elderly Cope Better with Belief in God. "

The Edmonton Journal, Jan. 13, 1994: "New $2.5 M. Residence to be Built for Victims of Alzheimer's Disease."

The Vancouver Sun, Nov. 1992: Pedersen, Rick, "Gardens Found to Soothe Alzheimer's Patients."

Van Manen, M. *Researching Lived Experience.* London, Ontario: Althouse Press, 1990.

Wiederkehr, Macrina, OSB. *A Tree Full of Angels.* San Francisco: Harper Collins Publishers, 1990.

Wilson, Paul. "Dementia: A Christian Response." *The Road To Greater Understanding.* CCOA Conference, April 24-25, 1992.

- - - - "Seniors Alive: The Challenge to the Religious Community and the Helping Professions." Proceedings of the Spiritual Well-Being of the Elderly Conference, Edmonton, Alberta. June, 1981.